Classic Comfort

Meghan Grey

Copyrights

28 Day *Instant Pot*

Rejuvenation

Menu:

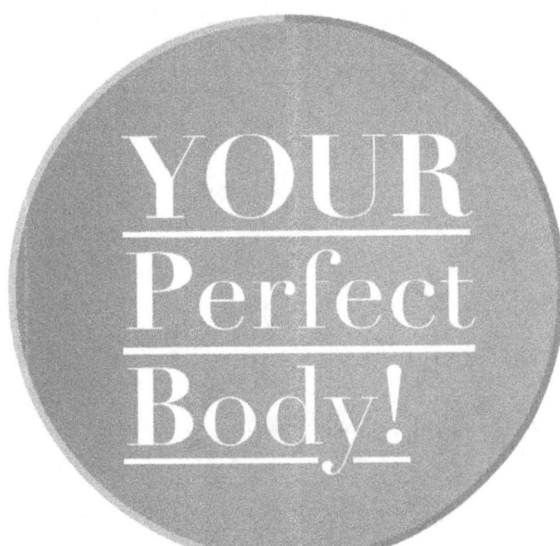

- *Breakfast*

- *Lunch*

- *Salad*

- *Dinner*

- *Dessert*

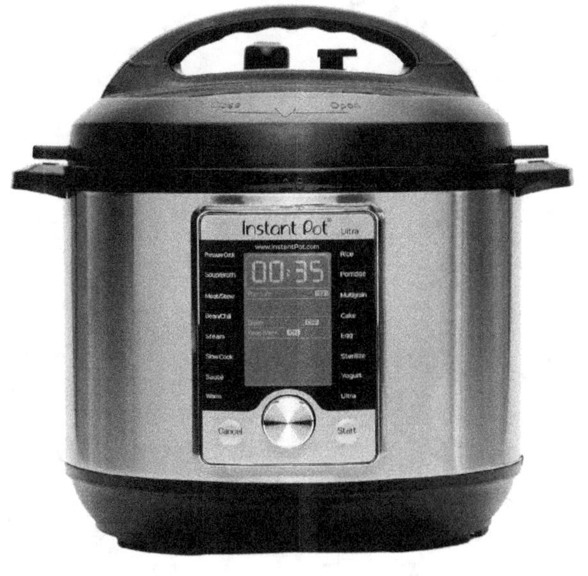

Table Of Contents:

Before you begin

A lmost all health problems are caused by either mental attitudes or physical inactivity, unhealthy eating habits and poor rest.

One of the main tools that will allow us to live a happy life is inside our head - this is our thinking. Only the realization that it is NOT effective for us, the desire to solve our problems and certainly the specific actions to solve them are the key to a healthy and HAPPY life. Only life in the present, not the past and the future, brings us really pleasure.

Remember how pleasant it is for you when you spend time with your friends, relatives, loved one or family. How you eat delicious food, how you watch an interesting movie, how you have a cool time on a long-awaited trip, and so on.

Or remember how fear and panic overwhelms you when you know that in a few days you will be thoroughly reprimanded at work or an unpleasant conversation will take place. At such a moment, you already feel bad, you have stress, but after all, a negative event has not happened yet, and you are already bad! Doesn't it seem strange to you? All of these examples show how we can be in the present with pleasure and in the future (without arriving in the present) under stress.

It's a good example of how psychology affects our health.

2020, the covid-19 epidemic began. The media only trumpets about deaths, negative consequences, complications, and political tensions. All this brings people into a state of fear and panic. In turn, this causes prolonged stress in people, and stress creates a hormonal background in the body that is responsible for catabolism, destruction processes. Long-term stress = excessive destruction of cells, primarily all cells responsible for immunity. In this way, a weakened immune system due to prolonged stress is less able to protect the body from pathogenic effects, which directly affects health. Immune barriers are weakened and bacteria and viruses(including covid-19) do their dark business with great ease, because weak immunity is no longer able to resist them. Moreover, the regeneration processes also slow down and it turns out that the destruction significantly prevails over the restoration of cells in the body = poor health, injury or even death. Also, all this is still influenced by poor nutrition, because our cells need specific substances that may not be enough in the diet of modern people.

«It is in your power to take your psychological and physical health under your control and be what you want, and not how it turns out.»

Follow the tips and recipes in this book, and in a month you will be amazed at how cool you have become. Big is small! Take a small step and go a long way.

The tips will be compiled by a very simple algorithm. It will be necessary to work on two aspects: on your thinking and on your physical health. Because the book is about food, here we will talk more about the physical aspects, but we will not miss the psychological ones, because this is also very important.

Some dishes take a long time to cook, due to the peculiarities of the multicooker and one or another dish. Therefore, some "breakfasts" should be started with dinner.
You need to look at the recipes for the next week in advance, since not all ingredients are everyday use and you will need to buy something.
The recipes in this book are not copyrighted or unique to this "menu plan". These are well-known recipes that have been selected for the purpose of developing a "menu" but not the recipes themselves. You may have met each of the dishes before.

How to get the best experience using this book:

Trying to follow the developed menu, at least 50%, will already be good. You can change each of the dishes for another, because it will not always be possible to cook the way it is written.
Carefully read the "recommendations" for each day, they were developed specifically for this book with the aim of improving your well-being.

Check the days that have passed, it will be better and more fun. You will be able to understand at what stage you are today and how much is still ahead.

Take everything easier and more fun. This book is not the ultimate true medical aid. This is a recovery menu, but if you ate your favorite dessert after 6:00 pm IT'S AWESOME!

(just kidding, once you can).

I hope you like my book and enjoy your time and open for yourself something new.

-with Love, Meghan Grey

I. GREEN WEEK

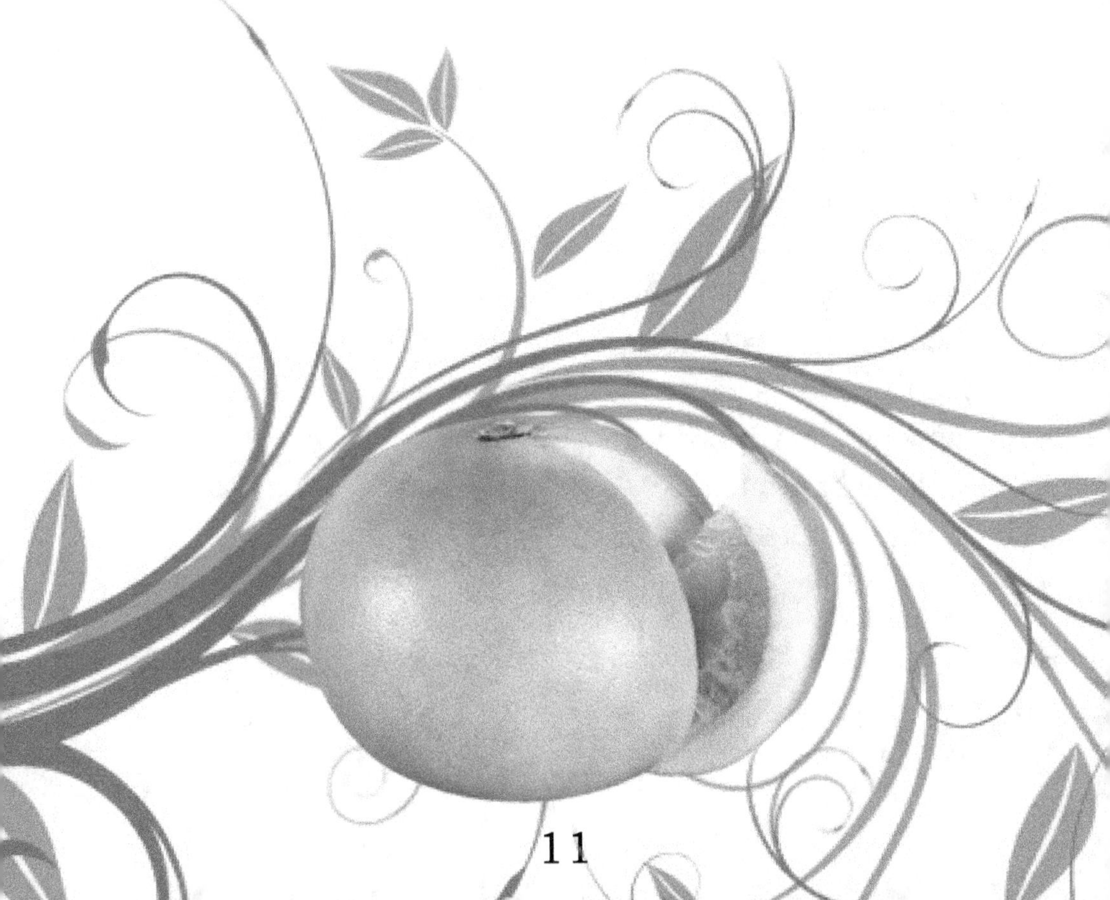

○ *DAY: 1*

RECOMMENDATION:

1. *The first thing I want to ask you to do for 1 month is to do the practice of gratitude. Every morning after you wake up, take a pen and notebook. Write down 10 thanks to yourself. What are you grateful to yourself for? It can be anything from small things to big accomplishments. This practice will improve your level of happiness, which will have a positive effect on your health.*

1. YOUR BREAKFAST:

Purple Yam Barley Porridge

Time - 45 m | **Servings** - 12

Ingredients:

3 tablespoons pearl barley

3 tablespoons pot barley

3 tablespoons buckwheat

3 tablespoons glutinous rice

3 tablespoons black glutinous rice

3 tablespoons black eye beans

3 tablespoons red beans

3 tablespoons romano beans

3 tablespoons brown rice

1 purple yam about 10.5 ounces

⅙ teaspoon baking soda optional

Directions:

1. Clean the purple yam, remove the skin and cut into 1 centimetre cubes.

2. Wash the barley, rice and beans in the inner pot of Instant Pot.

3. Place the purple yam and baking soda (if using) into the pot.

4. Add water up to the 8 cup mark on the inner pot.

5. Close the lid and put the steam release to the Sealing position. Select the [Porridge] program and keep pressing until the "More" setting is selected.

6. After the program finishes, let it cool for 10 minutes. Don't try to release the pressure as the starchy porridge will spill out.

7. Serve plain or with sugar, honey or blue agave syrup.

2. YOUR LUNCH:

Best Cabbage Soup, Ever

Time - 2 h | **Servings** - 5

Ingredients:

3 gold potatoes diced

2 large carrots diced

1 stalk celery diced

1 small yellow onion diced

½ head green cabbage chopped

14.5 ounce tomatoes diced, with juice, 1 can

2 Vegan Apple Sage Sausage links chopped

3 cups vegetable broth

1 ½ teaspoons salt

¼ teaspoon black pepper ground

Directions:

1. Place all the ingredients in the Instant Pot.

2. Cover with the lid and turn the lid clockwise to lock into place. Align the pointed end of the steam release handle to point to "Venting."

3. Press "Slow Cook", press "Adjust" to increase heat to "More", then use [-] button to adjust cooking time to 2 hours.

4. When time is up, open the lid of the Instant Pot.

5. Serve hot with whole grain bread rolls from your local bakery, or along with other dishes. Enjoy!

3. YOUR SALAD:

Superfood Salad

Time - 20 m | **Servings** - 6

Ingredients:

16 oz. shredded brussels sprout slow mix

2 pints fresh blueberries

1 medium green apple, diced into matchsticks

½ medium red onion, minced

1 cup cooked quinoa

1 cup golden raisins

1 cup slivered almonds

½ cup sunflower seeds

½ cup grapeseed oil (or olive oil)

2 teaspoons fresh grated ginger

1.5 tablespoons lemon juice

2 teaspoons apple cider vinegar

1 teaspoon honey

2 tablespoons fresh chopped parsley

2 tablespoon fresh chopped basil

¼ teaspoon ground turmeric

⅛ teaspoon salt

Pinch cayenne pepper

Directions:

1. Place all of the ingredients for the salad into a large salad bowl. Mix until combined and set aside.

2. Next, prepare the salad dressing by placing all ingredients for the dressing into a mason jar. Cover the mason jar and shake until all ingredients are combined.

3. Pour dressing over the salad and toss until everything is fully coated.

4. YOUR DINNER:

Hoisin-Glazed Baby Back Ribs

Time - 60 m | **Servings** - 6

Ingredients:

1 cup Hoisin Sauce

½ cup honey

1 tbsp Chinese five-spice powder

5 tbsp gochujang divided

2 tbsp minced fresh ginger

2 2 ½- to 3-lb racks baby back pork ribs each cut half if pressure cooking or cut into 3 or 4 rib sections if slow cooking

2 tbsp finely chopped fresh cilantro

2 tbsp sesame seeds toasted

3 scallions thinly sliced

Directions:

1. START: In a large bowl, whisk together the hoisin, honey, five-spice powder and 2 tbsp gochujang. Measure ¾ cup of the mixture into a small bowl and stir in the remaining 3 tbsp gochujang and the ginger; set aside at room temperature if pressure cooking or cover and refrigerate if slow cooking. Add the rib sections to the remaining hoisin mixture in the large bowl and turn to coat. Place the steam rack in a 6-quart Instant Pot, then pour in 1 cup water. Arrange the ribs upright in a circle, with the meaty sides facing the walls of the pot.

2. Fast (Pressure Cook): Lock the lid in place and move the pressure valve to Sealing. Select Pressure Cook or Manual; make sure the pressure level is set to High. Set the cooking

time for 25 minutes. When pressure cooking is complete, allow the pressure to reduce naturally for 15 minutes, then release the remaining steam by moving the pressure valve to Venting. Press Cancel, then carefully open the pot. Let cool for 5 minutes.

3. FINISH: While the ribs cool, heat the broiler with a rack about 6 inches from the element. Line a rimmed baking sheet with foil. Using tongs, carefully transfer the ribs meat side up to the prepared baking sheet. Generously brush with half of the reserved hoisin mixture and broil until the glaze begins to bubble, 2 to 3 minutes. Remove from the broiler, brush with the remaining mixture and continue to broil until bubbling, another 2 to 3 minutes. Cool for 5 minutes, then cut between the bones to separate into individual ribs. Transfer to a platter, then sprinkle with the cilantro, sesame seeds and scallions.

+ <u>YOUR DESSERTS</u>:

Cheesecake with Oreo

Time - 120 m | **Servings** - 6

Ingredients:

Cooking Spray

26 Oreos crushed, divided, plus more for garnish

3 tbsp melted butter

kosher salt

2 blocks cream cheese softened, 8 oz

½ cup granulated sugar

¼ cup packed brown sugar

¼ cup sour cream

2 large eggs

1 tsp pure vanilla extract

¼ tsp kosher salt

1 tbsp all-purpose flour

1 cup Water

Cool Whip for garnish

chocolate syrup for serving

Directions:

1. Make crust: Grease a 6 inch springform pan with cooking spray. In a medium bowl, combine 1 ½ cups crushed Oreos, melted butter, and a pinch of salt until mixture is the texture of wet sand.

2. Press mixture into bottom and up the side of the pan. Freeze for 20 minutes.

3. Meanwhile, make cheesecake: In a large bowl using a hand mixer, beat cream cheese, sugars, and sour cream until light and fluffy. Add eggs, one at time, and beat until just blended. Add vanilla, salt, and flour and beat until combined. Fold in remaining crushed Oreos. Pour batter on top of crust. Tightly wrap entire pan in two layers of foil.

4. Pour water into Instant Pot and place trivet in the bottom. Put springform pan on top. Secure lid and set to Pressure Cook on High for 37 minutes. Let pressure naturally release for 10 minutes, then follow manufacturer's guide for quick release, making sure to wait until cycle is complete before unlocking and removing lid.

5. Remove cheesecake from the pot, unwrap and discard foil, then place on a wire rack to cool for at least an hour. Refrigerate for 4 hours or overnight.

6. Garnish with Cool Whip, more Oreos, and chocolate syrup.

THANK YOU, GOOD JOB!

○ *DAY: 2*

RECOMMENDATION:

2. *The primary aspect in nutrition is enough water in your diet. In the case of water, it is better to drink heavily than not to drink. Excess water has almost no effect on the kidneys, while a lack of water severely wears out not only the kidneys, but the entire body. The skin dries faster, metabolic processes are worse and the body dies (gets old) faster. You don't have to look far for an example, look at homeless alcoholics who drink alcohol (which is a diuretic) and drink very little water. Such people in 25 may look 40-50 years old. Drink 10 or more glasses of water daily at any time.*

1. YOUR BREAKFAST:

Oatmeal, a Healthy Breakfast

Time - 20 m | **Servings** - 4

Ingredients:

2 cups rolled oats use gluten free if needed

4 cups Water

1 apple cored and diced

cinnamon to taste

Directions:

1. Place all ingredients in the Instant Pot and stir to combine.
2. Close and lock the lid. Use the "Rice" function to cook the oatmeal. When time is up, quick release the pressure.
3. Serve and Enjoy!

Creamy Curried Kabocha Squash Soup

Time - 20 m | **Servings** - 9

Ingredients:

8 cups Kabocha squash cooked

4 cups Water

¼ cup oats gluten free rolled

3 cups onion chopped

4-6 cloves garlic

1 tablespoon seasoning salt free or salted

2 teaspoons smoked paprika

1 teaspoon curry powder mild

¼ teaspoon ground ginger

¼ teaspoon ground turmeric

4 cups almond milk plain unsweetened

Directions:

1. Cook the squash according to your preferred method. The easiest way is to place the whole squash in the Instant Pot on the rack, filled with water up to the rack, and cook at high pressure for 10 minutes.
2. Remove carefully when cool enough to handle, cut squash in half and remove seeds.
3. Rinse out the pressure cooker insert to use again.
4. Place the seeded squash and all of the remaining ingredients, except for the almond milk, back into the insert and cook on high pressure for 5 minutes.
5. Release the pressure and add the almond milk. Using an immersion blender, add the almond milk and puree the soup right in the pot. Alternatively, carefully blend the contents in a blender.
6. This soup thickens as it cools so feel free to thin it out the next day with water or additional almond milk. Enjoy!

<u>3. YOUR SALAD:</u>

Kale with Edamame

Time - 20 m | **Servings** - 6

Ingredients:
1 bunch curly kale

stems and center rib removed and coarsely chopped

½ cup shelled edamame

½ cup grated carrots

¼ of a medium red onion, very thinly sliced

1 small red bell pepper, diced

½ ripe avocado, diced (I like to use a whole avocado, but I'm partial to avocado. You do you).

¼ cup roasted cashews, chopped

For the Miso Dressing:

1 tablespoon plus 1 teaspoon mellow white miso

1 clove garlic, pressed or finely grated

2 tablespoons fresh lime juice

2 teaspoons unseasoned rice vinegar

3 tablespoons extra virgin olive oil

1 teaspoon Sriracha

Directions:
1. Wash your kale very well and pat it dry. Remove the stems and center ribs from the kale. I just use my hands to do this, but you can use a knife if you prefer. Roughly chop the kale and transfer it to a large bowl.

2. Now it's time to prepare the miso dressing. Place all the ingredients for the miso dressing in a small bowl and whisk until well combined.

3. Pour ⅔ of the dressing over the kale and use your hands to rub the dressing into the kale leaves for about 3 minutes. This process is called "massaging the kale." It's kind of weird and annoying, but do NOT skip this step. This little massage will

make sure that your kale isn't tough and gross. Post-massage, set your kale aside for at least 15 minutes to marinate/tenderize.

4. While your kale is resting, prepare the rest of the ingredients for your salad. Add all of the ingredients except for the cashews to the massaged kale. Drizzle with the remaining miso dressing and toss to coat.

5. Sprinkle your kale salad with the chopped roasted cashews just before serving.

4. YOUR DINNER:

Honey Baked Ham

Time - 60 m | **Servings** - 6

Ingredients:

4 garlic cloves minced

4 tbs orange marmalade/jam

4 tbs Dijon mustard

3 tbs brown sugar

1 orange zested

1 cup Freshly Squeezed Orange Juice

1 tbs fresh rosemary

2 lb fully cooked smoked ham

Directions:

1. In a small bowl mix the garlic, orange marmalade (or jam), Dijon mustard, brown sugar, orange zest and orange juice. Use a hand blender to blend all the ingredients until you get a smooth glaze. Add the fresh thyme to the mixture.

2. Set your Instant Poti oven on Bake function at 360°F for 50 minutes. Place the ham on top of the baking pan and pour the glaze over the ham.

3. The ham is done when it is heated (the internal temperature should be ~145°F), and the glaze develops a golden-brown color.

Pumpkin Bread Pudding with Apple–Vanilla Sauce

Time - 120 m | **Servings** - 8

Ingredients:

Non-stick cooking spray

1 ½ cups 2% milk

2 eggs

¾ cup canned pumpkin

¼ cup sugar plus 1 tbsp sugar, divided

3 tbsp light butter with canola oil divided

1 tsbp Pumpkin Pie Spice

2 tsp vanilla extract divided

⅛ tsp salt

8 oz multigrain Italian loaf bread torn into small pieces

1 ¼ cups Water

1 sheet aluminum foil 18 inches long

¾ cup apple juice

1 ½ tsp cornstarch

Directions:

1. Coat a 7 inch nonstick springform pan with cooking spray.

2. Whisk together the milk, eggs, pumpkin, ¼ cup of the sugar, 2 tbsp of the light butter, the pumpkin pie spice, 1 tsp of the vanilla extract, and salt in a large bowl until well blended. Add the bread cubes and toss to coat well. Let stand for 10 minutes to allow the bread to absorb the milk mixture, stirring occasionally. Place the bread mixture into the springform pan; press down on the bread with the back of a spoon.

3. Place the water and a trivet in the Instant Pot. Cover the springform pan entirely with foil. Make a foil sling by folding an 18 inch-long piece of foil in half lengthwise. Place the pan in the center of the sling and lower the pan into the pot. Fold down the excess foil from the sling to allow the lid to close properly.

4. Seal the lid, close the valve, and set the Manual/Pressure Cook button to 40 minutes.

5. Use a natural pressure release for 10 minutes, followed by a quick pressure release. When the valve drops, carefully remove the lid. Remove the pan and sling carefully using the ends of the foil. Remove the foil from the springform pan. Let stand for 15 minutes to cool.

6. Meanwhile, remove the trivet and discard the water in the pot. Whisk together the apple juice and cornstarch in a small bowl. Press the Cancel button and set to Sauté. Then press the Adjust button to "More" or "High." Add the juice mixture and the remaining 1 tbsp of sugar to the pot. Bring to a boil and boil for 1 minute, or until thickened, stirring constantly. Remove the insert from the Instant Pot, and stir in the remaining 1 tbsp of light butter and 1 tsp of vanilla extract.

7. Cut the bread pudding into 8 wedges and serve topped with the sauce.

THANK YOU, GOOD JOB!

○ *DAY: 3*

RECOMMENDATION:

3. Set aside 5 minutes every morning for gymnastics. It can be some simple set of exercises or the simplest way: play your favorite music and dance actively. It will help you wake up and energize.

1. YOUR BREAKFAST:

Easy Vanilla Yogurt

Time - 20 m | **Servings** - 6

Ingredients:

4 cups milk 2%

3.5 ounces vanilla yogurt

1 tablespoon sugar

Directions:

1. Bring milk to boil in a medium size non-stick pot on high heat (option to do this in the Instant Pot by using the Saute function on high temperature).
2. Cool to near room temperature.
3. Add yogurt and sugar. Stir to mix. Divide the mixture into 4 heat proof cups. (If you used the Instant Pot for these steps, clean out the Instant Pot, it will be used in the following steps).
4. In the Instant Pot , add 5 cups water. Place the 4 heat proof cups into the inner pot. Close the lid and choose "Keep Warm" function for 15 minutes.
5. Let the pot stand for 10 hours closed.
6. Open the lid and take out yogurt. Cover with plastic wrap and chill a few hours before serving.

<u>2. YOUR LUNCH:</u>

Best Beef Bourguignon

Time - 30 m | **Servings** - 6

Ingredients:

4 slices bacon chopped

2 tablespoons butter or ghee, divided

24 white mushrooms wiped with damp cloth to clean, thinly sliced

½ teaspoon salt

¼ teaspoon pepper

1 ½ cups pearl onions frozen and defrosted or fresh and blanched and peeled

3 pounds lean sirloin 1-inch thick, trimmed and cubed into 1-inch pieces

6 tablespoons arrowroot

1 ½ cups burgundy wine

2 ½ cups beef bone broth

4 sprigs sage fresh

4 sprigs thyme fresh

Directions:

1. Set your Instant Pot to the Sauté setting. When display reads "hot", add the chopped bacon and cook until crisp.

2. Remove the bacon bits with a slotted spoon and set aside. Add 1 tablespoon of the butter/ghee and melt into the bacon drippings.

3. Add mushrooms to the pan and turn to coat evenly with butter and bacon drippings. Season with salt and pepper.

4. Sauté mushrooms for 2 to 3 minutes and add onions to the pan. Continue cooking onions and mushrooms 2 to 3 minutes longer, and then transfer to a plate.

5. With the setting still on sauté, add the remaining tablespoon of butter/ghee to the pan.

6. When melted, add meat and brown evenly on all sides. Add arrowroot to the browned meat and sauté for 2 minutes.

7. Slowly add wine to the pan while stirring. When the wine comes to a boil and you have scraped up the pan drippings, add the bone broth and herbs to the pot.

8. Return onions and mushrooms to the Instant Pot. Using the Manual setting, adjust the instant Pot to cook at high pressure for 12 minutes. When time is up, allow pressure to release naturally.

9. Remove the herbs and serve over cauliflower "rice" or cauliflower "mashed potatoes." Enjoy!

3. YOUR SALAD:

Spinach with Salmon

Time - 20 m | **Servings** - 6

Ingredients:

16 ounces smoked salmon, roughly chopped

2 avocado, peeled, pitted and diced

8 cups baby spinach

1 cup fresh blueberries

½ cup light feta or blue cheese crumbles

1 red onion, thinly sliced

honey chia seed vinaigrette

⅔ cup olive oil

4 tbsp. apple cider vinegar

2 tbsp. chia seeds

2 tbsp. honey

½ tsp. salt

Directions:

1. Toss all ingredients together until combined. Drizzle or toss with vinaigrette.

2. Whisk all ingredients together until combined and emulsified.

<u>4. YOUR DINNER:</u>

Awesome Slow Cooker Pot Roast

Time - 8 h | **Servings** - 12

Ingredients:
2 (10.75 ounce) cans condensed cream of mushroom soup
1 (1 ounce) package dry onion soup mix
1¼ cups water
5½ pounds pot roast

Directions:
1. In a slow cooker, mix cream of mushroom soup, dry onion soup mix and water. Place pot roast in slow cooker and coat with soup mixture.
2. Cook on High setting for 3 to 4 hours, or on Low setting for 8 to 9 hours.

<u>+ YOUR DESSERTS:</u>

Chia Berry Crepes

Time - 30 m | **Servings** - 3

Ingredients:
1 cup frozen blueberries

1 cup frozen raspberries

½ cup Water plus 1 tbsp of water, divided

2 tsp chia seeds

2 tsp cornstarch

3 tbsp powdered sugar divided

⅛ tsp almond extract

4 premade crepes

1 cup plain 2% Greek yogurt

Directions:

1. Place the berries, ½ cup of the water, and the chia seeds in the Instant Pot. Seal the lid, close the valve, and set the Manual/Pressure Cook button to 1 minute.

2. Use a quick pressure release. When the valve drops, carefully remove the lid.

3. In a small bowl, stir together the remaining 1 tbsp of water and the cornstarch. Stir until the cornstarch is dissolved.

4. Press the Cancel button and set to Sauté. Then press the Adjust button to "More" or "High." Stir the cornstarch mixture into the berries. Bring to a boil and boil for 1 minute, or until thickened slightly.

5. Turn off the heat. Stir in 2 tbsp of the powdered sugar and the almond extract. Place the berry mixture in a medium bowl and let stand for 15 minutes to cool slightly.

6. Spoon equal amounts of the berry mixture down the center of each crepe. Fold the ends over to overlap slightly. Spoon the remaining 1 tbsp of powdered sugar into a fine mesh sieve and sprinkle evenly over each crepe. Top each crepe with an equal amount of the yogurt. Serve warm or chilled, if desired.

THANK YOU, GOOD JOB!

○ *DAY: 4*

RECOMMENDATION:

4. Perform a total of 50 squats during the day. You can break it as you like. Do 5 sets of 10 squats, you can do 2 sets of 25 reps or whatever suits you best. Place your feet about one and a half shoulder-width apart, raise your arms in front of you and squat down until your thighs are parallel to the floor (90-degree knee angle). Make sure your back maintains physiological curves!

1. YOUR BREAKFAST:

Soy Milk Powder Yogurt

Time - 14 h | **Servings** - 5

Ingredients:

2 ½ cups hot water

¾ cup soy milk powder

1 teaspoon sugar

¾ teaspoon agar powder

¼ teaspoon probiotic or vegan starter culture

Directions:

1. Add water, soy milk powder and sugar to a high-speed blender. Blend for 3 minutes (The temperature will be around 166°F)

2. Add the agar powder and blend for 30 seconds longer (the temperature will now be around 172°F)

3. Allow the soy milk to cool down to 110°F (you can speed this process up by placing the blender carafe into a bowl of ice water).

4. Once the temperature is down to 110°F, add the probiotic powder or vegan culture and whisk into the soy milk (don't blend it)

5. Pour the soy milk into two 16-ounce glass jars.

6. Close the Instant Pot, set to sealing, and select the "yogurt" setting for 14 hours.

7. Remove the jars from the multi cooker, cover with lids, and allow to cool on the counter before storing in the refrigerator. Though firm out of the Instant Pot, this is best served after two or more hours in the refrigerator. Enjoy!

2. YOUR LUNCH:

Hungarian Beef Stew

Time - 30 m | **Servings** - 6

Ingredients:

1 ½ pounds lean chuck roast boneless, trimmed and cut into 1 inch pieces

¾ teaspoon table salt

½ teaspoon black pepper freshly ground

2 tablespoons olive oil

2 medium onions chopped

1 tablespoon paprika

1 teaspoon caraway seeds

3 cloves garlic minced

1 cup dry red wine & 1 ¾ cups Water

1 ½ cups beef stock unsalted

1 pound fingerling potatoes cut into 1 inch chunks

3 carrots coarsely chopped

2 red bell peppers sliced

2 tablespoons all-purpose flour

Directions:

1. Sprinkle beef with ½ teaspoon of the salt and ¼ teaspoon of the pepper.

2. Remove the lid from a 6-quart Instant Pot. Press Sauté. When the word "Hot" appears, swirl in oil.

3. Add one-third of beef to inner pot; cook 5 minutes or until golden brown on both sides. Transfer to a plate with a slotted spoon. Repeat procedure with remaining beef in 2 additional batches.

4. Add onions; cook, stirring constantly, 5 minutes or until softened. Add paprika, caraway seeds, and garlic; cook 1 minute, stirring. Add wine; cook 2 minutes, stirring occasionally and scraping brown bits from bottom of pot. Add 1 ½ cups of the water, remaining ¼ teaspoon salt and remaining ¼ teaspoon pepper, stock, and beef, with accumulated juices, to the pot.

5. Close and lock the lid of the Instant Pot. Turn the steam release handle to "Sealing" position. Cook at High Pressure 25 minutes. Allow a 10-minute Natural Pressure Release. Turn steam release handle to "Venting" to release remaining pressure.

6. Turn cooker off, and remove lid. Add potatoes, carrots, peppers. Close and lock the lid of the Instant Pot. Turn the steam release handle to "Sealing" position. Cook at High Pressure 5 minutes. Open the cooker using Quick Pressure Release. Turn cooker off.

7. Gradually add the remaining ¼ cup water to the flour, stirring until smooth; add to stew, stirring constantly. Press Sauté, and select "Less" mode. Cook, stirring frequently, 5 minutes or until stew boils and thickens slightly.

8. Serve and enjoy!

<u>3. YOUR SALAD:</u>

Tuna and Bean
Time - 10 m | **Servings** - 4

Ingredients:
6 cups arugula

22.5 ounces cannellini beans, rinsed and drained

7.5 ounces white albacore tuna packed in water, drained

0.75 cup cherry tomatoes, halved

0.38 cup sliced olives

Thinly sliced red onion & 0.75 lemon

3 tablespoons extra virgin olive oil

0.38 cup crumbled feta cheese

Kosher salt and freshly ground black pepper

Directions:
1. In a large bowl or two smaller bowls, combine the arugula, white beans, tuna, tomatoes, olives and and red onion.
2. Drizzle with the olive oil and the juice from the lemon. Toss to combine.
3. Top with crumbled feta cheese and season to taste with kosher salt and black pepper.

<u>4. YOUR DINNER:</u>

Parmesan Roast Chicken with Lemon
Time - 60 m | **Servings** - 6

Ingredients:
2 lemons small

3 tsp kosher salt plus more to taste

3 tsp black pepper

2 tsp rosemary chopped

6 rosemary sprigs

2 tsp red pepper flakes plus more for serving, optional

1 whole chicken about 3 pounds

extra-virgin olive oil for drizzling

⅓ cup parmesan finely grated

4 cups chicken stock

Directions:

1. Finely grate 2 teaspoons of zest from the lemons and place into a small bowl. (Save the zested lemon for the drippings.)

2. Stir in 3 teaspoons salt, pepper, chopped rosemary and red-pepper flakes (if using). Season the chicken inside and out with salt mixture and set aside. Stuff cavity of chicken with 2 rosemary springs.

3. Place the chicken breast-side down, add the chicken, the stock, and 2 of the rosemary springs into the inner pot. Place the inner pot into your Instant Pot and select Pressure Cook, and set to High pressure for 20 minutes.

4. When pressure cooking is complete, Quick Release the pressure.

5. Remove the lid, using tongs take the chicken out of the inner pot and drain the water.

6. Making sure that your inner pot is dry, place the air fryer basket (or trivet) into the pot, drizzle the chicken with the olive oil and place it into the basket.

7. Using the Air fryer Lid select Roast at 400°F for 25 minutes. In the middle of the cooking process sprinkle the chicken with the parmesan cheese. Continue roasting.

8. When cooking is complete the internal temperature should reach 165°F. Let the chicken rest for 5 to 10 minutes then squeeze juice from one of the zested lemons over the chicken.

9. Carve and serve drippings spooned over the meat.

Chocolate and Banana Chip Cake

Time - 120 m | **Servings** - 8

Ingredients:

½ cup coconut oil room temperature & 1 cup monk fruit sweetener

2 large eggs room temperature

3 medium bananas mashed & 2 cups oat flour

1 ½ tsp baking soda & ½ tsp salt

½ cup stevia-sweetened chocolate chips

Directions:

1. In a large bowl of a stand mixer with a paddle attachment, add the oil, sweetener, and eggs and beat together on medium speed until well combined.
2. Add the mashed banana and beat until combined.
3. Add the flour, baking soda, and salt and beat again until combined.
4. Remove the paddle attachment and stir in the chocolate chips.
5. Spray a 6 inch Bundt cake pan with cooking oil. Transfer the batter into the pan. Place a paper towel over the top of the pan and then cover with aluminum foil.
6. Add 1 ½ cups water to the Instant Pot inner pot and then place a steam rack inside. Place the Bundt pan on the steam rack. Secure the lid.
7. Press the Manual or Pressure Cook button and adjust the time to <strong<="" strong="">. </strong
8. When the timer beeps, let pressure release naturally for 10 minutes, then quick-release any remaining pressure until float valve drops, then unlock lid.
9. Allow to cool completely before removing from pan and slicing to serve.

THANK YOU, GOOD JOB!

○ *DAY: 5*

<u>RECOMMENDATION:</u>

5. *If it seems to you that it is difficult to eat right and lead an active lifestyle, then this is not so. If you start everything gradually, then after 6 months you can achieve fantastic results and the new way of life will be a pleasure.*

<u>1. YOUR BREAKFAST:</u>

Slow Cook Steel-Cut Oatmeal with Apples

Time - 6 h | **Servings** - 10

Ingredients:

4 cups Granny Smith apple diced, about 1 pound

2 cups steel cut oats gluten-free, such as Bob's Red Mill

7 cups Water

½ cup honey or liquid sweetener of choice (maple syrup or agave to make it vegan), adjust to preference of sweetness

½ teaspoon salt

½ teaspoon allspice ground

13.6 ounce coconut milk light, 1 can

cashews toasted, optional

Granny Smith apple diced for topping, optional

Directions:

1. Coat the inner pot of the Instant Pot with oil. Combine apple and next 6 ingredients (oats through coconut milk) in inner pot.
2. Close and lock the lid of the Instant Pot. Turn the steam release handle to "Venting" position. Press [Slow Cook], and use [Adjust] to select "Less" mode. Press [-] or [+] to choose 6 hours cook time.

3. Stir well before serving. Garnish with toasted cashews and additional diced apple, if desired. Enjoy!

2. YOUR LUNCH:

Smokey Cheesy Split Pea Soup

Time - 20 m | **Servings** - 5

Ingredients:

3 medium potatoes peeled, halved

3 stalks celery chopped

1 large carrot chopped

1 small yellow onion chopped

2 cloves garlic chopped

2 cups green split peas dried, rinsed

1 teaspoon liquid smoke

1 teaspoon marjoram dried

1 teaspoon basil dried

1 bay leaf

1 teaspoon sea salt

⅛ teaspoon ground black pepper

1 cup Thick & Creamy Nacho Cheese Sauce recipe in the app

Water enough to cover all ingredients in the Instant Pot by 1 inch

Directions:

1. Place all the ingredients in the inner pot. Cover all ingredients with enough to have 1 inch of water standing over all ingredients.

2. Cover with lid, turn lid clockwise to lock into place. Align the pointed end of the steam release handle to point to "Sealing." Press "Manual", use [-] button to adjust cooking time to 10 minutes.

3. When cooking time is complete, press "Keep Warm/Cancel" once to cancel the keep warm mode then wait 10 minutes for the pressure to go down.

4. Slide the steam release handle to the "Venting" position to release remaining pressure until the float valve drops down. Remove lid.

5. Remove bay leaf.

6. Use an immersion blender to puree soup. Stir in Thick & Creamy Nacho Cheese Sauce. This recipe is located in the app under side dishes for the full recipe.

7. Serve hot with whole grain dinner rolls. Enjoy!

3. YOUR SALAD:

Avocado Caprese

Time - 10 m | **Servings** - 2

Ingredients:

2 cups fresh arugula

2-3 campari or cocktail style tomatoes sliced

½ avocado pitted and sliced

3 slices fresh mozzarella cheese

fresh basil leaves

1 tablespoon extra virgin olive oil I prefer the fruitiest, lightest flavored

1 ½ teaspoons balsamic vinegar

generous pinch of sugar or dollop of honey

kosher salt and freshly ground black pepper

Directions:

1. Assemble the arugula, tomato, avocado slices and mozzarella in a serving bowl. Top with torn or slivered basil leaves. Whisk the extra virgin olive oil in a small bowl with the balsamic vinegar, sugar or honey and season with kosher salt and freshly ground black pepper to taste and pour over the salad. Toss to coat and serve.

<u>4. YOUR DINNER:</u>

Italian-Style Braised Pork Chops

Time - 30 m | **Servings** - 4

Ingredients:

1 cup chicken broth

2 tbsp balsamic vinegar

2 tsp stemmed thyme leaves or 1 tsp dried thyme

¼ tsp grated fresh nutmeg or ⅛ tsp ground nutmeg

¼ tsp red pepper flakes

¼ tsp table salt

4 cups frozen bell pepper strips 16-ounce bag

4 frozen center-cut boneless pork loin chops 6- 8-ounce each

Directions:

1. Stir the broth, vinegar, thyme, nutmeg, red pepper flakes, and salt in an Instant Pot. Mix in the frozen pepper strips, then set the pork chops in the pot so they stand up on their sides and lean against each other and the side of the insert with room between each for liquid and pepper strips (in other words, not in a stack). Lock the lid onto the pot.
2. Option 1 Max Pressure Cooker
3. Press Pressure cook on Max pressure for 16 minutes with the Keep Warm setting off.
4. Optional 2 All Pressure Cookers
5. Press Meat/Stew, Pressure Cook or Manual on High pressure for 20 minutes with the Keep Warm setting off. The vent must be closed.
6. Use the quick-release method to bring the pot's pressure back to normal. Unlatch the lid and open the cooker. Transfer the pork chops to serving plates and spoon some of the sauce and peppers over each .

Cream Cheesecake & Cookies

Time - 120 m | **Servings** - 6

Ingredients:

1 cup Water

26 cream-filled chocolate sandwich cookies divided

2 tbsp unsalted butter melted

16 oz cream cheese softened

½ cup granulated sugar

1 tsp vanilla extract

½ cup full-fat sour cream

2 large eggs room temperature

Directions:

1. Pour water into Instant Pot and add trivet. Grease a (7 inch) push pan and set aside.

2. Place 16 chocolate cookies in a gallon-sized zip-top bag and seal. Roll with a rolling pin until small crumbs are formed.

3. In a small bowl, mix crushed cookies and melted butter together.

4. Press cookie crust into bottom and halfway up sides of greased PushPan. Place pan in freezer while preparing cheesecake batter.

5. With an electric mixer, cream together cream cheese, sugar, and vanilla. Beat until light and fluffy, about 2 minutes.

6. Slowly mix in sour cream and mix.

7. Add eggs one at a time, beating after each addition Only mix until combined. Do not overmix.

8. Chop remaining cookies and fold half of them into cheesecake batter. Reserve remaining chopped cookies for topping.

9. Pour batter into the push pan. Create a foil sling and carefully lower pan into Instant Pot.

10. Close lid and set pressure release to Sealing.

11. Press Manual or Pressure Cook button and adjust time to 40 minutes.

12. When the timer beeps, allow pressure to release naturally and then unlock lid and remove it.

13. Carefully remove pan from Instant Pot using foil sling. Place on a cooling rack and let cool to room temperature.

14. Cover with plastic wrap and refrigerate for a minimum of 8 hours.

15. Top cheesecake with remaining chopped cookies and serve.

THANK YOU, GOOD JOB!

○ *DAY: 6*

RECOMMENDATION:

6. My advice to someone maybe too radical, but 2 hours before bedtime, I recommend not to use any electronic devices, not to read books, not to engage in active physical and intellectual activity. And also dim the lighting in the room by 50%. This will make it easy to fall asleep and recuperate efficiently.

1. YOUR BREAKFAST:

Slow Cook Maple French Toast Casserole

Time - 90 m | **Servings** - 8

Ingredients:

Cooking Spray

12 slices sandwich bread cut into 1 inch pieces, can use gluten free bread

4 eggs lightly beaten

½ cup maple syrup

1 teaspoon cinnamon & ½ teaspoon salt

¼ teaspoon nutmeg grated

⅛ teaspoon cloves ground

2 cups milk reduced fat 2%

1 teaspoon powdered sugar

Directions:

1. Coat the inner pot of the Instant Pot with cooking spray.
2. Place cubed bread in the pot
3. Combine eggs, maple syrup, cinnamon, salt, cloves and nutmeg in a large bowl.

4. Add milk, stirring with a whisk until blended. Pour milk mixture over bread in the pot, pressing gently with a spoon to coat all bread pieces.

5. Tear off a 10 ½ inch long piece of aluminum foil; lay foil on top of inner pot, gently smoothing it down the side of the pot. trim pointed corners even with rest of the foil, and tightly tuck it under the rim

6. Cut 2 (1 ¼ inch long) slit in the foil about one inch from the edge with a thin sharp knife. Cut a second slit parallel to and about 1 inch to the inside of the first. Repeat this procedure 3 times, creating 2 concentric slits in foil at intervals of 12, 3, 6, and 9 o'clock.

7. Set inner pot inside cooker. Close and lock the lid of the Instant Pot. Turn steam release handle to Venting. Select the Slow Cook function and adjust time to 90 minutes cooking time.

8. Serve warm sprinkled with powdered sugar. Enjoy!

2. YOUR LUNCH:

Split Pea Soup with Mushrooms

Time - 10 m | **Servings** - 8

Ingredients:

1 pound green split peas

1 large onion chopped

1 pound carrots sliced

1 heart celery sliced

2 large potatoes cubed

8 cups Water boiling

2 cups sundried tomatoes oil free, chopped

8 ounces cremini mushrooms dried

6-8 cloves garlic pressed

4 teaspoons dried parsley

1-2 tablespoons salt-free seasoning

1 teaspoon dried basil

1 teaspoon dried rosemary

1 teaspoon dried oregano

1 teaspoon celery seed

1 teaspoon smoked paprika

1 bay leaf

Directions:

1. Place all ingredients in the Instant Pot.

2. Cook on high pressure for 8 minutes by pressing Manual function and adjusting to high pressure. Alternately, cook on slow cook function and cook on low for 6-8 hours.

3. When time is up allow for natural pressure release.

4. Serve over brown rice and/or raw or cooked spinach or other greens. Or stir in some greens right after releasing the pressure. Enjoy!

3. YOUR SALAD:

Detox Salad

Time - 100 m | **Servings** - 5

Ingredients:

2 large sweet potatoes

6 cups kale, chopped

2 cups red cabbage, thinly sliced

1 yellow squash, chopped

⅓ cup apple cider vinegar

⅓ cup lemon juice & ⅓ cup tahini

1 tablespoon honey

1 tablespoon ginger, minced

1 clove garlic, minced

2 tablespoons cilantro, chopped

salt to taste (I used 1 teaspoon sea salt).

Directions:

1. Bake sweet potatoes until tender.
2. Allow to cool enough to handle and then dice. Refrigerate until cold.
3. Bring a large pot of water to a boil.
4. Add the kale to the water just until it turns bright green (about 1 minute). Drain.
5. Refrigerate kale until cold.
6. Combine all vegetables, adding the sweet potatoes last and being careful not to mash them.
7. Whisk together remaining ingredients until well combined.
8. Pour over the vegetables and toss to coat.

4. YOUR DINNER:

Coconut-Curry Rice and Vegetable

Time - 60 m | **Servings** - 6

Ingredients:

⅔ cup uncooked brown rice rinsed and drained & 1 cup Water

1 tsp curry powder & ¾ tsp salt divided

1 cup chopped green onion both green and white parts

1 cup sliced red or yellow bell pepper

1 cup matchstick carrots

1 cup chopped red or purple cabbage

1 can sliced water chestnuts drained, 8 oz

1 can no salt added chickpeas rinsed and drained, 15 oz

1 can lite coconut milk 13 oz

1 tbsp grated fresh ginger & 1 ½ tbsp sugar

Directions:

4. Combine the rice, water, curry powder, and ¼ tsp of the salt in the Instant Pot.
5. Seal the lid, close the valve, and set the Manual/Pressure Cook button to 15 minutes.

6. Use a natural pressure release for about 12 minutes. When the valve drops, carefully remove the lid and stir in the remaining ingredients.

7. Press the Cancel button and set to Sauté. Then press the Adjust button to "More" or "High." Bring to a boil and boil for 2 minutes, or until all the ingredients are heated through, stirring occasionally.

+ YOUR DESSERTS:

Steel Cut Baked Oatmeal Bars with Raspberry

Time - 60 m | **Servings** - 6

Ingredients:

3 cups steel cut oats & 3 large eggs

2 cups unsweetened vanilla almond milk

⅓ cup erythritol & ¼ tsp salt

1 cup frozen raspberries & 1 tsp pure vanilla extract

Directions:

1. In a medium bowl, mix together all ingredients except the raspberries. Once the ingredients are well combined, fold in the raspberries.

2. Spray a 6" cake pan with cooking oil. Transfer the oat mixture to the pan and cover the pan with aluminum foil.

3. Pour 1 cup water into the Instant Pot and place the steam rack inside. Place the pan with the oat mixture on top of the rack. Secure the lid.

4. Press the Manual or Pressure Cook button and adjust the time to 15 minutes.

5. When the timer beeps, quick-release pressure until float valve drops and then unlock lid.

6. Carefully remove the pan from the inner pot and remove the foil. Allow to cool completely before cutting into bars and serving.

THANK YOU, GOOD JOB!

RECOMMENDATION:

7. *Sign up for some kind of sports section for general physical development. For example, fitness, yoga, running, swimming, active games, etc.*

1. YOUR BREAKFAST:

Classic Irish Oatmeal

Time - 30 m | **Servings** - 5

Ingredients:

2 tablespoons butter

1 cup steel cut oats & 3 cups Water

½ teaspoon salt

½ teaspoon ground cinnamon

⅓ cup half and half

¼ cup brown sugar packed

1 cup strawberries quartered

6 ounces blackberries & 6 ounces blueberries

3 tablespoons granulated sugar & 1 tablespoon Water

Directions:

1. Press Saute; melt butter in Instant Pot. Add oats; cook about 5 minutes, stirring frequently.
2. Add water, salt and cinnamon; cook and stir 1 minute.
3. Secure lid and move pressure release valve to Sealing position. Select Manual; cook at high pressure 13 minutes.
4. Meanwhile, prepare Berry Compote, if desired.
5. When cooking is complete, press Cancel to turn off heat. Use natural release for 10 minutes, then release remaining pressure.

6. Stir oats until smooth. Add half-and-half and brown sugar; stir until well blended.

7. If a thicker porridge is desired, press Sauté and cook 2 to 3 minutes or until desired thickness, stirring constantly. (Porridge will also thicken upon standing). Serve with Berry Compote.

To Make the Compote

8. Combine 1 strawberries, blackberries, blueberries, granulated sugar and 1 tablespoon water in medium saucepan; bring to a simmer over medium heat.

9. Cook 8 to 9 minutes or until berries are tender but still hold their shape, stirring occasionally.

2. YOUR LUNCH:

Wholesome Veggie Pasta Soup

Time - 40 m | **Servings** - 6

Ingredients:

2 stalks celery diced

1 large carrot diced

1 small yellow onion diced

1 small red bell pepper diced

2 teaspoons dried parsley

1 bay leaf

6 cups vegetable broth

28 ounce kidney beans rinsed and drained, 2 cans

1 ½ cups pasta dry

3 cups baby spinach fresh

1 cup mushrooms sliced

⅛ teaspoon black pepper ground

Directions:

1. Press the "Sauté" button; add celery, carrot, onion, bell pepper, dried parsley, bay leaf and ¼ cup vegetable broth.

2. Sauté vegetables in broth until onions are translucent, about 8 minutes. If the inner pot becomes dry before onion is tender, add 2 tablespoons broth to prevent vegetables from sticking.

3. Add remaining broth, kidney beans, pasta, spinach, mushrooms, and pepper.

4. Continue to simmer soup until pasta is tender to the bite, 10 to 15 minutes, depending on pasta type.

5. Remove bay leaf. Press "Keep Warm/Cancel" twice to activate keep warm mode.

6. Serve right away or cover with lid, the soup is ready when your family is ready to eat. Enjoy!

3. YOUR SALAD:

Marinated Vegetables

Time - 30 m | **Servings** - 5

Ingredients:

1 head of garlic

2 tbsp fresh thyme leaves

1 tbsp fresh rosemary leaves

8 fresh bay leaves

1 tbsp Maldon salt

2-3 tsp cracked black peppercorns (these can be bought in jars)

150ml/¼ pint olive oil

900g/1.3kg/2-3lb of assorted vegetables (e.g. asparagus, large or baby courgettes, sweet potatoes, aubergines, fennel, red onions, corn cobs, parboiled new potatoes)

Directions:

1. Peel the garlic cloves and tip into a food processor with the thyme, rosemary, bay leaves, salt, peppercorns and oil. Whizz well to release the flavours – alternatively grind dry ingredients using a pestle and mortar then blend in the oil.

2. Prepare 900g-1.3kg/2-3lb of assorted vegetables (e.g asparagus, large or baby courgettes, sweet potatoes,

aubergines, fennel, red onions, corn cobs, parboiled new potatoes). Halve asparagus lengthways, cut large courgettes into chunks or halve baby ones lengthways. Cut sweet potatoes and aubergines into thick chunks, cut fennel and red onion lengthways into wedges, corn into chunks and potatoes in half lengthways. Mix the vegetables and marinade together and marinate for a couple of hours before barbecuing. Cooking times will vary according to your choice of vegetables and their thickness – keep turning and prodding them and you'll feel when they're done.

4. YOUR DINNER:

Spinach and Feta Stuffed Chicken

Time - 30 m | **Servings** - 4

Ingredients:

4 boneless, skinless chicken breasts butterflied (6 ounce

½ cup frozen spinach & ⅓ cup crumbled feta cheese

1 ¼ tsp salt divided & ¼ tsp pepper

¼ tsp garlic powder

¼ tsp dried oregano & ¼ tsp dried parsley

2 tbsp coconut oil & 1 cup Water

Directions:

1. Pound chicken breasts to ¼-inch thickness. In medium bowl, mix frozen spinach and feta and add ¼ teaspoon salt. Evenly divide mixture and spoon onto chicken breasts.

2. Close chicken breasts and secure with toothpicks or butcher's string. Sprinkle remaining seasonings onto chicken. Press the Sauté button and add coconut oil to Instant Pot. Sear each chicken breast until golden brown (this may take two batches). Press the Cancel button.

3. Remove chicken and set aside briefly. Pour water into Instant Pot and scrape bottom to remove any chicken or seasoning that is stuck on. Place steam rack into pot.

4. Place chicken on steam rack and click lid closed. Press 'Pressure Cook' and adjust time for 15 minutes. When timer beeps, allow a

15-minute natural release, then quick-release the remaining pressure. Serve warm with favorite white sauce if desired.

<u>+ YOUR DESSERTS:</u>

Mixed Berry Mousse

Time - 120 m | **Servings** - 4

Ingredients:

20 oz thawed frozen blackberries (4 cups) blueberries & raspberries

6 tbsp sugar divided

1 tsp finely grated lemon zest & Pinch table salt

1 ½ tsp unflavored gelatin & ½ cup heavy cream

3 oz cream cheese softened

Directions:

1. Combine berries, 3 tablespoons sugar, lemon zest, and salt in bowl and let sit for 30 minutes, stirring occasionally.

2. Strain berries through fine-mesh strainer over separate bowl; transfer berries to Ace blender and set aside. Transfer 3 tablespoonsdrained juice into small bowl, sprinkle gelatin over top, and let sit until gelatin softens, about 5 minutes. Meanwhile, microwave remaining juice until reduced to 3 tablespoons, 4 to 5 minutes. Whisk gelatin mixture and remaining 3 tablespoons sugar into reduced juice until dissolved.

3. Lock blender lid in place, then process berries on Medium speed until smooth, about 30 seconds. Add gelatin mixture, heavy cream, and cream cheese to blender, return lid, and process on medium speed until combined, about 10 seconds. Increase speed to High and process until smooth, about 30 seconds, pausing to scrape down sides of blender jar as needed.

4. Portion mousse into 4 individual serving dishes. Cover with plastic wrap and refrigerate until set, at least 4 hours or up to 2 days. Serve.

<u>THANK YOU, GOOD JOB!</u>

II. *YELLOW WEEK*

8 9 10 11 12 13 14

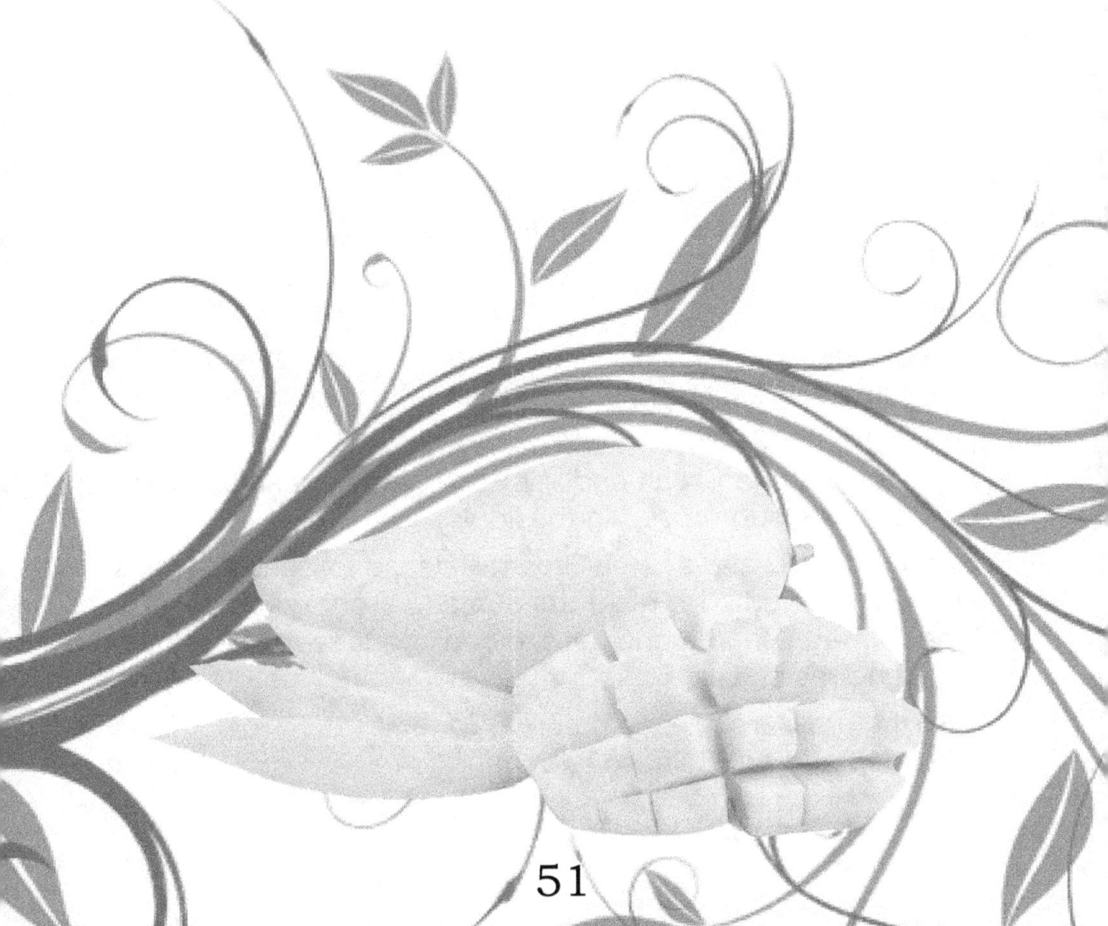

○ *DAY: 8*

RECOMMENDATION:

8. A healthy spine is an important part of health. And since the majority are now sedentary and sedentary, the spine needs special attention. Perform 3 sets of crunches for the press and bending back (extensions) for the back, about 20-30 times daily.

1. YOUR BREAKFAST:

Brown Butter Steel-Cut Oatmeal

Time - 20 m | **Servings** - 6

Ingredients:

2 tablespoons unsalted butter

1 ½ cups steel cut oats

4 ½ cups Water

½ teaspoon kosher salt

brown sugar for serving & heavy cream for serving

Directions:

1. Select Saute on the Instant Pot and melt the butter. Add the oats and sauté, stirring often, for about 5 minutes, until aromatic and lightly toasted.
2. Add the water and salt and stir to combine, making sure all of the oats are submerged in the liquid.
3. Secure the lid and set the Steam Release to Sealing. Press the Cancel button to reset the cooking program, then select the Porridge setting and set the cooking time for 12 minutes at high pressure.
4. Let the pressure release naturally for at least 10 minutes, then move the Steam Release to Venting to release any remaining

steam. Open the pot and stir the oatmeal to incorporate any extra liquid.

5. Ladle the oatmeal into bowls and serve with brown sugar and cream.

2. YOUR LUNCH:

Chicken Soup

Time - 40 m | **Servings** - 6

Ingredients:

2-3 pounds chicken

2 carrots roughly chopped

1 celery roughly chopped

¼ Turnip or Radish, cut in 2 inch cubes

1 tablespoon Italian seasoning or ½ teaspoon each of dried parsley, oregano, thyme and rosemary

2 bay leaves & 3 cloves garlic crushed

1 piece Ginger thumb sized sliced

1 medium onion sliced

1 tablespoon sea salt

1 teaspoon black pepper fresh ground

scallion thinly sliced, for garnish

purple onion thinly sliced, for garnish

Directions:

1. In the inner pot, add the vegetables first, then, chicken, and the herbs on top.

2. Add 4 cups of cold water.

3. Close the lid tightly and close the vent. Press Soup function on the Instant Pot.

4. When the timer goes off, release the pressure naturally. It may take about 20-30 minutes after the timer goes off for the vent to open.

5. Open the lid, take out the chicken and de-bone the meat.

6. Reserve the bones to make bone broth. Put the meat back to the pot and stir.

7. Crush the carrots and celery gently against the side of the pot with the back of a spoon.

8. Add salt and pepper to taste.

9. Garnish with thinly sliced onions, and scallions to serve. Enjoy!!

3. YOUR SALAD:

Bean & Cheese

Time - 10 m | **Servings** - 5

Ingredients:

290g jar artichoke heart in oil

1 tbsp sundried tomato paste

1 tsp white wine vinegar

410g can cannellini beans, drained and rinsed

300g pack small vine tomato, quartered (about 12 in total)

handful Kalamata black olives

2 spring onions, thinly sliced on the diagonal

200g log soft goat's cheese, crumbled

Directions:

1. Drain the jar of artichokes, reserving 3 tbsp of the oil. Pour the oil into a bowl and stir in the sun-dried tomato paste and vinegar until smooth. Season to taste.

2. Roughly chop the artichokes and tip into a large bowl with the cannellini beans, tomatoes, olives, spring onions and half the goat's cheese. Stir in the artichoke oil mixture and tip into a serving bowl. Season to taste. Crumble over the remaining goat's cheese, then serve.

<u>4. YOUR DINNER:</u>

Easy Chicken Noodle Soup

Time - 60 m | **Servings** - 4

Ingredients:

½ lbs boneless skinless chicken breasts

1 carrot peeled and chopped (about ½ cup)

1 stalk celery sliced (about ½ cup)

2 oz uncooked extrawide egg noodles about 1 cup dry

4 cups Chicken Broth

Directions:

1. Season the chicken with salt and pepper. Add the carrot, celery, chicken, noodles and broth to a 6 quart Instant Pot.

2. Lock the lid and close the pressure release valve. Pressure cook on High pressure, setting the timer to 5 minutes (timer will begin counting down once pressure is reached- it takes about 15 minutes). When done, press Cancel and use the quick release method to release the pressure.

3. Remove the chicken from the pot. Shred the chicken and return to the pot. Season to taste.

<u>+ YOUR DESSERTS:</u>

Mango and Sticky Rice

Time - 60 m | **Servings** - 4

Ingredients:

1 cup Thai sticky rice sweet rice, or glutinous rice

1 ⅓ cups canned full-fat coconut milk well stirred

7 tbsp organic cane sugar

½ tsp fine sea salt or kosher salt plus more to taste

1 tbsp cornstarch

2 ripe Ataúlfo mangoes peeled, pitted, and thinly sliced or diced, honey, about 6 ounces each

2 tbsp yellow mung beans toasted, or 2 teaspoons toasted white sesame seeds or black sesame seeds

Directions:

1. For easy removal of the pan from the Instant Pot, create a foil sling. (Alternatively, you can use oven mitts to carefully remove the pan.)

2. Place the sticky rice in a large bowl and add water to cover. Gently stir the rice with your hands, then drain the water, and repeat 4 or 5 times until the water runs almost clear. This removes the excess starch and prevents the rice from becoming gummy. Place the rinsed rice in a heatproof glass or stainless steel bowl that fits inside the inner pot of your Instant Pot. Add ⅔ cup cold water to the bowl to cover the rice.

3. On the counter, place the bowl on top of the steamer rack with the handles facing up and arrange the foil sling (if using) underneath the steamer rack. Pour 1 ½ cups water into the inner pot of the Instant Pot. Carefully lower the steamer rack and bowl into the inner pot using the foil sling or steamer rack handles.

4. Secure the lid and set the Pressure Release to Sealing. Select the Pressure Cook setting at high pressure and set the cook time to 13 minutes.

5. Once the 13-minute timer has completed and beeps, allow a natural pressure release for 10 minutes and then switch the Pressure Release knob from Sealing to Venting to release any remaining steam.

6. While the pot is depressurizing, in a small saucepan, bring ⅔ cup of the coconut milk to a simmer over medium heat. Add 5 tbsp of the cane sugar and ¼ tsp of the salt and whisk until the sugar is dissolved and the milk tastes salty-sweet. Keep the sauce warm.

7. Open the Instant Pot and, with oven mitts, transfer the cooked sticky rice to a large bowl and pour the warm coconut milk mixture on top. Stir well to combine and gently fluff with a fork. Cover and let it sit until the liquid is absorbed, about

20 minutes. You can let the rice rest at room temperature for up to 2 hours.

8. Meanwhile, set aside 2 tbsp of the remaining coconut milk in a small bowl. Wipe out the saucepan and add the remaining coconut milk. Add the cornstarch to the small bowl and whisk until smooth, forming a slurry. Bring the coconut milk in the saucepan to a simmer over medium heat, whisking frequently. Whisk the slurry into the coconut milk on the stove and simmer until the mixture has thickened, about 2 minutes. Whisk in the remaining 2 tbsp cane sugar and the remaining ¼ tsp salt until the sugar is dissolved. The coconut cream should be slightly saltier and less sweet than the coconut milk mixture used to cover the rice.

9. When ready to serve, use a 1-cup measuring cup to scoop the coconut rice into mounds on individual plates and arrange the sliced or diced mango alongside. Drizzle the warm coconut cream over the rice and garnish with the toasted yellow mung beans or sesame seeds. Serve immediately. Do not warm up or refrigerate, as the rice will turn rock hard.

THANK YOU, YOU'RE DOING FINE!

○ *DAY: 9*

<u>RECOMMENDATION:</u>

9. Walk as often as possible and preferably in places far from traffic so that there is clean air around. This has a very positive effect on health.

1. YOUR BREAKFAST:

Perfectly Cooked Eggs

Time - 10 m | **Servings** - 3

Ingredients:

1 cup Water

1-6 eggs large or jumbo

Directions:

1. Pour the water into the Instant Pot. Place a steamer basket or the trivet in the pot.
2. Carefully arrange eggs in the steamer basket. Secure the lid on the pot. Close the pressure-release valve.
3. For soft-cooked eggs, select manual and cook at low pressure for 3 minutes. When cooking time is complete, use a natural release to depressurize. (For medium-cooked eggs, cook for 4 minutes; for hardcooked eggs, cook for 5 minutes).
4. Remove the lid from the pot and gently place eggs in a bowl of cool water for 1 minute to serve warm.

Plant Based Butternut Ginger Bisque

Time - 10 m | **Servings** - 5

Ingredients:

1 cup yellow onion diced

4 cloves garlic minced

2 teaspoons Ginger peeled and chopped

1 cup carrot chopped

1 green apple chopped (discard the core and seeds)

1 butternut squash peeled and chopped (about 4 cups)

1 teaspoon salt

2 cups Water

¼ cup parsley finely chopped

black pepper

Directions:

1. Prep and measure out all of the ingredients before you start.

2. Press the saute button on your Instant Pot and heat for 2 minutes. Add the onions and cook for 5 minutes, adding a splash of water when they start to stick or look dry.

3. Add the garlic, ginger, carrot, apple, squash and salt and stir. Turn off the Instant Pot and add the water. Lock the lid into place, making sure the nozzle is in the sealing position.

4. Use the manual setting and set the timer for 5 minutes. When the timer goes off, use the natural release method. When all the pressure is out of the Instant Pot, take off the lid and allow to cool for about 15 minutes.

5. In batches, blend the soup in your blender (or all in one go with a blender stick) until all of the soup is blended and it's super creamy and smooth.

6. Add the parsley and black pepper and stir. Enjoy!

<u>3. YOUR SALAD:</u>

Tomato with Herbs & Feta

Time - 20 m | **Servings** - 4

Ingredients:

6 to 7 medium ripe tomatoes (on-the-vine tomatoes or heirloom tomatoes preferred), sliced into wedges

1 medium red onion, halved, then thinly sliced

3 garlic cloves, minced

1 packed cup chopped fresh parsley leaves

1 packed cup chopped fresh dill

2 ½ tsp ground sumac

Salt and freshly ground pepper

1 lemon, juice of

2 tsp white wine vinegar

⅓ cup Early Harvest Greek extra virgin olive oil

Feta cheese, optional

Directions:

1. In a large salad or mixing bowl, add the tomatoes, onions, fresh herbs and garlic. Add sumac, salt and a generous sprinkle of freshly ground pepper.
2. Add the lemon juice, white wine vinegar, and extra virgin olive oil. Toss well to combine. Taste and adjust the salt to your liking.
3. Transfer to a serving platter or bowl. Top with large slices of quality feta cheese (optional). Enjoy!

<u>4. YOUR DINNER:</u>

Pot Roast

Time - 120 m | **Servings** - 6

Ingredients:

2 ½ lbs boneless beef chuck roast (up to 3 lbs

1 tbsp vegetable oil

½ cup dry red wine

2 large Onions cut into large chunks or wedges (about 3 cups)

5 large carrots peeled and cut into 2 inchpieces or2 ½ cups of baby cut carrots

1 lbs whole baby red potatoes or medium red potatoes cut in half

2 sprigs fresh thyme leaves

1 can Condensed Cream of Mushroom Soup 10 ½ ounces

Directions:

1. Cut the beef in half crosswise (for quicker cooking), then season with salt and pepper. On a 6 quart Instant Pot, select the Saute setting. Heat the oil. Add the beef (in batches, if needed) and cook for 15 minutes or until well browned on all sides. Remove the beef from the pot. Add the wine and cook, stirring to scrape up the browned bits from the bottom of the pot. Press Cancel.

2. Layer the onions, carrots, potatoes, thyme and beef in the Instant Pot. Spoon the soup over the beef (the order is important, so don't stir until after the cooking is done).

3. Lock the lid and close the pressure release valve. Pressure cook on High pressure, setting the timer to 45 minutes (timer will begin counting down once pressure is reached- it takes about 10 minutes). When done, press Cancel and use the quick release method to release the pressure.

4. Remove the beef to a serving plate, cover and keep warm. Select the Saute setting and cook the vegetables and gravy for 10 minutes or until the gravy is slightly thickened. Remove

and discard the thyme. Season to taste. Slice the beef and serve with the vegetables and gravy.

+ YOUR DESSERTS:

Cherry Pie Brandy-Soaked Cheater

Time - 60 m | **Servings** - 6

Ingredients:

2 lbs cherries pitted

⅓ cup brandy

⅔ cup sugar

3 tbsp cornstarch

pinch salt

½ juice of lime

3.8 oz mini fillo shells (2 boxes 1.9 oz each)

Directions:

1. In a large bowl, combine the cherries and brandy. Let soak for 30 minutes, stirring occasionally.

2. On your Instant Pot, select Sauté Low. When the display reads "Hot," pour the cherries and whatever liquid is at the bottom of the bowl into the inner pot. Stir in the sugar, cornstarch, salt, and lime juice. Cook for 10 to 15 minutes, stirring frequently so nothing burns, until thickened.

3. Let cool for a few minutes before spooning the filling into the fillo shells.

THANK YOU, YOU'RE DOING FINE!

○ <u>*DAY: 10*</u>

<u>RECOMMENDATION:</u>

10. There is such a thing as species food. This is what the animal should eat according to the idea of nature. Cows, for example, have different grasses, birds have worms and seeds, frogs have insects. The people also have the own specific food, which gives them health, this is primarily vegetables and fruits. Therefore, try to eat as much as possible of various fresh vegetable salads and fruits.

<u>1. YOUR BREAKFAST:</u>

Breakfast Hash

Time - 40 m | **Servings** - 5

Ingredients:

3 tbsp butter

1 medium yellow onion chopped (1 cup)

1 medium green bell pepper stemmed, cored, and chopped (1 cup)

1 medium red bell pepper stemmed, cored, and chopped (1 cup)

1 lb smoked deli ham (not thinly shaved), any coating removed, the meat diced

2 medium garlic cloves peeled and minced (2 teaspoons)

1 tsp dried sage & 1 tsp dried thyme

½ tsp celery seeds (optional)

¼ tsp fine table salt

¼ tsp ground black pepper

1 lb yellow potatoes diced (no need to peel)

1 ½ cups chicken broth

Directions:

1. Press Saute, set time for 5 minutes.

2. Melt the butter in a the cooker. Add the onion and both bell peppers. Cook, stirring occasionally, until softened, about 4 minutes. Add the ham, garlic, sage, thyme, celery seeds (if using), salt, and pepper. Cook, stirring often, until fragrant, about 1 minute.

3. Turn off the SAUTE function. Stir in the potatoes and broth, scraping up any browned bits on the pot's bottom. Lock the lid onto the cooker.

4. Optional 1 Max Pressure Cooker

5. Press Pressure cook on Max pressure for 10 minutes with the Keep Warm setting off.

6. Optional 2 All Pressure Cookers

7. Press Pressure cook (Manual) on High pressure for 12 minutes with the Keep Warm setting off.

8. Use the quick-release method to bring the pot's pressure back to normal. Unlatch the lid and open the cooker. Stir well.

9. Press Saute, set time for 10 minutes.

10. Bring the mixture to a simmer, stirring often. Continue without stirring until the liquid boils off and the hash touching the hot surface starts to brown, 3 to 4 minutes. Turn off the SAUTE function and remove the hot insert from the machine to stop the cooking. Some of the potatoes may have fused to the surface. Use a metal spatula to get them up. The point is to have some browned bits and some softer bits throughout the hash.

2. YOUR LUNCH:

Oxtail Ragout

Time - 40 m | Servings - 6

Ingredients:

2 tablespoons butter or ghee

1 large onion diced & 2 stalks celery diced

2 carrots peeled and diced & 1 ½ cups beef bone broth

14 ounces tomatoes diced, 1 can & 2 bay leaves

1-2 teaspoons thyme fresh or ½ -1 teaspoon dried

½ teaspoon rosemary fresh, or ½ teaspoon dried

½ teaspoon salt & 3 peppercorns

3 oxtails joints separated, about 4 pounds

2 teaspoons red wine vinegar

2 tablespoons arrowroot (optional)

2 tablespoons Water (optional)

Directions:

1. Set your Instant Pot to the Sauté setting. When display reads "hot", heat the butter/ghee and sauté the onions, celery, and carrots for 2 minutes, or until softened.
2. Add beef bone broth, tomatoes, bay leaves, thyme, rosemary, salt, and peppercorns and stir.
3. Add in the oxtails.
4. Using the Manual setting on the Instant Pot, adjust to high pressure and set to cook for 30 minutes. When time is up, allow pressure to naturally release.
5. Skim off any excess fat, remove the bay leaves and peppercorns and add the red wine vinegar.
6. If you wish to thicken the ragout, blend the arrowroot into 2 tablespoons of water. Bring the ragout to a boil on the Sauté setting and stir in the arrowroot mixture.
7. Boil gently, stirring constantly until the ragout has thickened, about 2 minutes. Serve and enjoy!

3. YOUR SALAD:

Mango & Tuna

Time - 20 m | **Servings** - 3

Ingredients:

4 tablespoons vegetable oil & 1 mango diced in large chunks

2 tablespoon ponzu sauce & 1 teaspoon prepared wasabi

8 ounces sushi grade tuna diced in large chunks

1 cup store-bought seaweed salad

1 teaspoon black sesame seeds

4-6 cups loosely packed spring lettuce mix & 1 avocado sliced

½ teaspoon pink Hawaiian sea salt

Directions:

1. In a small bowl, whisk the vegetable oil, ponzu sauce and wasabi until well blended.

2. Add the tuna, mango and seaweed salad to a bowl and drizzle with 1 tablespoon or so of the dressing. Sprinkle with the sesame seeds and stir to coat.

3. In a different bowl, add the lettuce and avocado and top with the tuna mixture. Drizzle with more dressing as desired and sprinkle with Hawaiian sea salt and more sesame seeds. Serve immediately.

4. YOUR DINNER:

Bean and Sausage Soup

Time - 60 m | **Servings** - 6

Ingredients:

½ lbs Italian-style chicken sausage casing removed

1 extra large onion diced (about 1 ½ cups)

2 cloves garlic minced & 2 tbsp olive oil

1 can white cannellini beans rinsed and drained, about 15 ounces

1 tsp Italian seasoning & 4 cups Chicken Broth

3 cups packed finely chopped kale leaves trim leaves from stems before chopping

2 tbsp grated parmesan cheese

Directions:

1. On a 6 quart Instant Pot, select the Saute setting. Heat the oil. Add the sausage and cook for 10 minutes or until well browned, stirring often to separate meat. Press Cancel.

2. Add the onion, garlic, beans, Italian seasoning and broth. Lock the lid and close the pressure release valve. Pressure

cook on High pressure, setting the timer to 3 minutes (timer will begin counting down once pressure is reached- it takes about 10 minutes). When done, press Cancel and use the quick release method to release the pressure.

3. Stir in the kale and let stand for 5 minutes. Season to taste and sprinkle with the cheese.

+ YOUR DESSERTS:

Apple Pie

Time - 20 m | **Servings** - 6

Ingredients:

3 ½ lb assorted sweet and tart apples

2 tsp lemon juice freshly squeezed & 2 tsp ghee

¼ tsp ground cinnamon plus more for serving

⅛ tsp ground allspice & ⅛ tsp fine sea salt

Directions:

1. Peel, core, and slice the apples. Place the apples, ¾ cup water, and the lemon juice, ghee, cinnamon, allspice, and salt in an electric pressure cooker.

2. If using an Instant Pot, secure the lid and turn the valve to pressure. Select the Manual or Pressure Cook button and set it to high pressure for 5 minutes.Once the timer has sounded, let the machine release the pressure on its own; it will take about 15 minutes. (Alternatively, carefully release the pressure manually.) Remove the lid.

3. Using an immersion blender or conventional blender, pulse the applesauce to your desired consistency. Serve warm with cinnamon sprinkled on top, or refrigerate and enjoy chilled.

4. Store the applesauce in an airtight container in the refrigerator for 10 days or in an airtight container in the freezer for 6 months. Allow it to thaw overnight in the refrigerator before serving. If desired, reheat in a saucepan over medium-low heat for 8 to 10 minutes, until heated through.

THANK YOU, YOU'RE DOING FINE!

○ _DAY: 11_

RECOMMENDATION:

11.As often as possible, go on vacation to nature. Firstly, it helps the psyche to calm down, because we are one with nature and returning to it, we get tranquility. And secondly, clean air, which fills the cells of the body with energy.

1. YOUR BREAKFAST:

Classic Deviled Eggs

Time - 20 m | **Servings** - 6

Ingredients:

6 large eggs

¼ cup mayonnaise

1 tsp mustard

¼ tsp salt

¼ tsp pepper

Smoked paprika and chopped chives for garnish

Directions:

1. Place the Instant Pot steam rack in the Instant Pot inner pot and add 1 cup of water. Place the eggs on top of steam rack (you can also use a steamer basket instead of the steam pot). Secure the lid, ensuring the valve is turned to the Sealing position. Press the Pressure Cook button and set the time to 7 minutes.

2. When cooking is complete, turn the valve to the Venting position to release the pressure. Remove the lid and remove the eggs with a pair of tongs. Place the eggs in a bowl and fill it with cool water until the eggs are cool enough to handle. Peel the eggs under running water, pat them dry, and then slice the eggs in half lengthwise.

3. Remove the egg yolks from the whites and place them in a medium bowl, reserving the whites. Add the mayonnaise, mustard, and the salt and pepper to the yolks and mix well. Spoon the egg-yolk mixture back into the egg white halves and sprinkle the tops with smoked paprika and chopped chives. Serve the eggs cold or at room temperature.

2. YOUR LUNCH:

Fast Tasty Rice

Time - 15 m | **Servings** - 7

Ingredients:

1 ½ pounds asparagus

2 pounds sweet potatoes orange or white

6 cups vegetable broth low sodium, or water

1 large onion

8 cloves garlic

2 tablespoons dried dill

2 tablespoons salt-free seasoning

3-4 cups nondairy milk unsweetened, adjust amount depending on desired thickness

4 tablespoons Dijon mustard or stone ground mustard

4 tablespoons nutritional yeast optional

Directions:

1. Place all ingredients except for the plant milk, mustard and nutritional yeast (if using), in the Instant Pot.
2. Select Manual function and cook on high pressure for 6 minutes. When time is up, release pressure.
3. Add the almond milk, mustard and nutritional yeast.
4. Puree with an immersion blender right in the pot until smooth.
5. This soup is delicious served over black, red or wild rice, or alone.

<u>3. YOUR SALAD:</u>

Greek Salad

Time - 15 m | **Servings** - 4

Ingredients:

1 green bell pepper, cored

1 medium red onion

4 Medium juicy tomatoes, preferably organic tomatoes

1 Cucumber, or ¾ English (hot house) cucumber preferred, partially peeled making a striped pattern

Greek pitted Kalamata olives

Salt, a pinch

4 tbsp quality extra virgin olive oil (I used Early Harvest Greek olive oil)

1–2 tbsp red wine vinegar

Blocks of Greek feta (do not crumble) a good amount to your liking

½ tbsp quality dried oregano

Directions:

1. Cut the tomatoes into wedges or large chunks (I sliced some and cut the rest in wedges).
2. Cut the partially peeled cucumber in half lengthwise, then slice into thick halves (at least ½" in thickness)
3. Thinly slice the bell pepper into rings.
4. Cut the red onion in half and thinly slice into half moons.
5. Place everything in a large salad dish. Add a good handful of the pitted kalamata olives.
6. Season very lightly with salt (just a pinch). Pour the olive oil and red wine vinegar.
7. Give everything a very gentle toss to mix; do NOT over mix, this salad is not meant to be handled too much.
8. Now add the the feta blocks on top. Sprinkle the dried oregano.
9. Serve with crusty bread.

Shrimp Gumbo

Time - 60 m | **Servings** - 6

Ingredients:

¼ cup vegetable oil

¼ cup all-purpose flour

4 stalks celery chopped

1 large yellow onion peeled and diced

1 large green bell pepper seeded and diced

2 garlic cloves peeled and minced

1 can diced tomatoes 14.5 ounce

¼ tsp dried thyme

¼ tsp cayenne pepper

2 bay leaves

1 tbsp filé powder

2 tsp Worcestershire sauce

4 cups Seafood Stock

1 lb smoked sausage sliced

1 lb medium shrimp peeled and deveined

¼ tsp salt

¼ tsp ground black pepper

2 cups cooked long-grain rice

Directions:

1. Press the Sauté button on the Instant Pot and heat oil. Add flour and cook, stirring constantly, until flour is medium brown in color, about 15 minutes.

2. Add celery, onion, green pepper, garlic, and tomatoes and cook, stirring constantly, until the vegetables are tender, about 8 minutes. Add thyme, cayenne, bay leaves, filé, Worcestershire sauce, and stock and stir well, making sure nothing is stuck to the bottom of the pot, then add sausage. Press the Cancel button.

3. Close lid and set steam release to Sealing, then press the Manual button and adjust cook time to 8 minutes. When the timer beeps, quick release the pressure. Open lid and stir in shrimp, salt, and black pepper. Press the Cancel button, then press the Sauté button and cook for 8 minutes, or until shrimp are cooked through. Discard bay leaves. Serve hot over rice.

+ YOUR DESSERTS:

Vanilla-Scented Rice Pudding

Time - 30 m | **Servings** - 6

Ingredients:

¼ teaspoon sea salt

¼ teaspoon cinnamon

¼ cup brown sugar

1 whole vanilla bean split along one side

3 cups arborio or short-grain white rice

¾ cup raisins

For cooking and serving

4 ½ cups Water

½ cup heavy cream or coconut cream

Directions:

1. Layer the dry ingredients in the jar in the order listed.

2. Place all of the jarred ingredients into the Instant Pot. Add 4 ½ cups of water. Stir tomix. Cover with the lid and ensure the vent is in the "Sealed" position. Pressure Cook or Manual on High for 8 minutes. Allow the steam pressure to release naturally for 10 minutes, then release any remaining pressure manually. Stir in the heavy cream or coconut cream and allow to rest for 5 minutes before serving.

THANK YOU, YOU'RE DOING FINE!

○ *DAY: 12*

RECOMMENDATION:

12.Everyone knows about hygiene? To wash your hair, brush your teeth, wash your hands ... But few people know that the insides should also be washed. I'm talking about the esophagus, stomach and intestines. And this washing is done by simply drinking water after waking up. During the night without moving, bacteria multiply in the mouth and esophagus and should be removed. You can rinse your mouth, and brush your teeth, but you can't rinse deeper (esophagus, intestines). Therefore, you need to wash off everything with clean water. This is a simple morning hygiene routine. In addition, drinking water will help to start up intestinal motility and make it easy to go to the toilet.

1. YOUR BREAKFAST:

Sous Vide - Avocado Toast with Poached Egg

Time - 45 m | **Servings** - 4

Ingredients:

4 eggs

2 avocados

2 tbsp olive oil

fresh lime juice

4 slices whole grain bread toasted

fresh basil leaves chopped

Freshly cracked black pepper

sea salt

Directions:

1. Preheat a water bath to 145°F. Bring a pot of water to a boil on the stovetop. Prepare an ice bath with half ice and half water. Gently place the eggs in the boiling water and cook for 3 minutes.

2. Remove from the boiling water and place in the ice bath for 1 to 2 minutes, then transfer to the water bath. Let the eggs cook for 45 minutes. Once cooked, remove them from the water bath.

3. Peel and remove the flesh from the avocado, and mash together with the olive oil. Add the lime juice, and salt and pepper to taste, until the spread is slightly tangy and well balanced.

4. Take a slice of toasted bread and slather on some of the avocado spread. Crack a poached egg on top slather on some of the avocado spread. Crack a poached egg on top then sprinkle with the basil, fresh cracked pepper, and sea salt.

2. YOUR LUNCH:

Spicy Butternut Stew

Time - 20 m | **Servings** - 6

Ingredients:

3 cups vegetable broth & 1 cup yellow onion chopped

2 cups butternut squash cut into small cubes

2 cups kidney beans cooked, rinsed and drained

1 cup yellow corn kernels fresh or frozen & 2 cloves garlic minced

14.5 ounce diced tomatoes 1 can & 1 teaspoon paprika

1 teaspoon ground cumin

⅛ teaspoon Ancho chili powder

Directions:

1. Place all the ingredients in the inner pot. Cover with lid, turn lid clockwise to lock into place. Align the pointed end of the

steam release handle to point to "Sealing." Press "Manual", use [-] button to adjust cooking time to 5 minutes.

2. When cooking time is complete, press "Keep Warm/Cancel" once to cancel the keep warm mode then wait 10 minutes for the pressure to go down.

3. Slide the steam release handle to the "Venting" position to release remaining pressure until the float valve drops down.

4. Remove lid. Allow to cool 10 minutes before serving. Enjoy!

3. YOUR SALAD:

Mediterranean Vegetables

Time - 10 m | **Servings** - 5

Ingredients:

1 large red bell pepper, thinly sliced

1 large carrot, cut on diagonal into ½-inch slices

¼ lb. white mushrooms, halved

1 ½ cups coarsely chopped plum tomatoes

⅓ cup pitted oil-cured black olives

1 ½ tsp. dried basil leaves

1 ½ tsp. dried oregano leaves

1 tsp. salt or to taste & ¼ tsp. cinnamon

⅛ tsp. freshly ground pepper

1 to 3 Tbs. balsamic vinegar or lemon juice

1 Tbs. olive oil & 2 tsp. minced garlic

1 cup coarsely chopped onions

1 small fennel bulb, cut into ½-inch strips (about 2 ½ cups; chop and reserve fronds)

Directions:

1. In large skillet, heat oil over medium heat. Add garlic and onions and cook, stirring often, until just browned, about 5 minutes. Add fennel bulb, bell pepper, carrot, mushrooms, tomatoes, olives, basil, oregano, salt, cinnamon and pepper.

2. Reduce heat, cover and simmer until vegetables are tender,
    about 4 minutes. Add vinegar, stir well and cook 1 minute.

3. Serve over couscous if desired, and garnish with reserved
    fennel fronds.

4. YOUR DINNER:

Mongolian Beef

Time - 30 m | **Servings** - 6

Ingredients:

1 ½ pounds flank or sirloin steak thinly sliced

2 tbsp corn starch & 1 package spices for meat to taste

2 tbsp oil & 1 cup Water

¾ cup reduced-sodium soy sauce & ⅓ cup packed brown sugar

2 green onions cut into 1 inch pieces, green parts only

Directions:

1. Place beef in large resealable bag. Add corn starch; close bag
    tightly and shake to coat beef. Heat oil in Instant Pot
    on SAUTÉ setting. Add beef to pot; cook and stir 3 minutes.
    Remove beef from pot. Add water; stirring with whisk to
    remove browned bits from bottom of pot. Stir in brown sugar,
    soy sauce and Seasoning Mix until well blended. Return beef
    to pot. Close lid. Set Valve to Seal.

2. Select PRESSURE COOK (MANUAL); cook 7
    minutes on HIGH PRESSURE. When done, quick-
    release pressure. Open lid once pressure inside pot is
    completely released. (Check manufacturer's manual for safe
    operating instructions.) Stir in green onions.

+ YOUR DESSERTS:

Chocolate Yogurt

Time - 120 m | **Servings** - 12

Ingredients:

23 oz ultra-filtered chocolate milk like Fairlife

1 tbsp plain or vanilla yogurt with active cultures

Directions:

1. Pour one cup of water in the Instant Pot and insert the steam rack. On the rack place tools that need to be sterilized: a 1-cup glass measure containing a 1 tbsp measure and a heatproof silicone spatula.
2. Using the display panel select the STEAM function. Use the +/- keys and program the Instant Pot for 3 minutes.
3. When the time is up, quick-release the pressure. Allow to cool, then remove the tools without touching the inside of the pot or any other surface that will touch food. Drain the pot without touching the inside of the pot.
4. Using the sterilized tbsp measure, add 1 tbsp of the active-culture yogurt to the sterilized glass measure. Add ⅔ cup of the milk to the glass measure and use the sterilized spatula to stir until smooth.
5. Add the remainder of the milk and the yogurt mixture to the pot and use the sterilized spatula to stir until all yogurt is incorporated, then secure the lid, making sure the vent is closed.
6. Choose the YOGURT function and adjust to the NORMAL or MEDIUM setting. Use the +/- keys and program the Instant Pot for 8 hours.
7. At the end of the 8 hours, cover the inner pot with plastic wrap and refrigerate at least 8 hours. Do not stir at this point.
8. At the end of the refrigeration time you will have a pourable chocolate yogurt that pairs wonderfully with fresh berries and granola for a delicious breakfast treat.
9. To make yogurt pops, pour yogurt mixture into popsicle molds and freeze for at least 8 hours. Unmold and enjoy.

THANK YOU, YOU'RE DOING FINE!

○ *DAY: 13*

RECOMMENDATION:

13.From time to time arrange fasting days for yourself. It can be done once every 7 days, or less often. Eat ONLY vegetable salads and fruits these days. This will allow the digestive system to rest, which is the prevention of diseases such as type 2 diabetes mellitus, gastritis, duodenitis and other gastrointestinal diseases.

1. YOUR BREAKFAST:

Sous Vide - Apple-Cinnamon Oatmeal

Time - 30 m | **Servings** - 1

Ingredients:

⅔ cup Bob's Red Mill Organic Quick Cook Steel Cut Oats

¼ cup diced apples

1 ⅓ cups Water

¼ tsp ground cinnamon

dash of salt

maple syrup

Almond slivers

Thinly sliced apple

Directions:

1. Preheat a water bath to 183°F.
2. Combine the oats, apple, water, cinnamon, and salt in a pint (16 ounce) jar. Screw the lid on the jar until it's finger-tight, basically until you feel medium resistance when tightening using only your fingertips.
3. This will allow some air to escape during the sous vide process and help prevent breakage.

4. Shake the jar, then carefully place it in the water bath. Cook the oatmeal for 30 to 45 minutes, until the water is absorbed and the oatmeal is cooked through, shaking the jar once or twice during the process.

To Assemble

5. Spoon the oatmeal into a bowl. Drizzle with maple syrup, then top with almond slivers and apple slices.

2. YOUR LUNCH:

5 Minute Vegetable Stew

Time - 20 m | Servings - 6

Ingredients:

1 bell pepper chopped

1 medium yellow onion chopped

1 jalapeno fresh, seeds removed, minced

14.5 ounce tomatoes diced with juice, 1 can

4 cups canary beans or pinto beans, cooked and drained

1 cup corn fresh or frozen

1 tablespoon chili powder

1 ½ teaspoons ground cumin

1 cup cilantro fresh, chopped

1 ½ cups vegetable broth

Directions:

1. Place all the ingredients in the inner pot.

2. Cover with lid, turn the lid clockwise to lock into place. Align the pointed end of the steam release handle to point to "Sealing." Press "Manual", use [-] button to adjust cooking time to 4 minutes.

3. When cooking time is complete, press "Keep Warm/Cancel" once to cancel the keep warm mode then wait 10 minutes for the pressure to go down.

4. Slide the steam release handle to the "Venting" position to release remaining pressure until the float valve drops down. Remove lid.

5. Serve hot with fresh baked cornbread. Enjoy!

3. YOUR SALAD:

Cabbage Rolls

Time - 40 m | **Servings** - 4

Ingredients:

1 large head green cabbage

2 Tbs. coconut oil

2 parsnips, diced

2 garlic cloves, minced

½ cup walnuts, toasted and chopped

3 cups chopped mushrooms of any variety

2 carrots, diced

Sauce

½ cup Dijon mustard

¼ cup honey or agave

1 Tbs. walnut oil

2 Tbs. minced tarragon

⅓ cup finely chopped flat leaf parsley

Directions:

1. Bring a large pot of salted water to a boil. Using a sharp paring knife, cut the core out of the cabbage. Carefully lower the whole head of cabbage into the boiling water, and cook for 4 to 5 minutes, until outer leaves begin to loosen. Remove cabbage from water and carefully peel off 8 outer leaves. Reserve remaining cabbage for another use.

2. In a large skillet, heat coconut oil and sauté mushrooms, carrots, and parsnips until tender, 4 to 5 minutes. Add garlic and cook for 1 minute longer, stirring. Stir in walnuts. Remove from heat and let cool slightly.

3. To assemble, place one cabbage leaf on a flat surface. Mound a few spoonfuls of filling in the center of leaf. Fold bottom of leaf over filling, and roll up about ⅓ of the way. Fold sides in and continue rolling into a tight roll. Place on a platter, seam side down. Repeat with remaining rolls and filling.

4. To make sauce: Whisk together mustard, honey or agave, walnut oil, and tarragon in a small bowl. Season to taste with salt and pepper. Drizzle over cabbage rolls, shower with parsley, and serve.

4. YOUR DINNER:

Beer Cheese Soup

Time - 60 m | **Servings** - 8

Ingredients:

3 tbsp unsalted butter

2 medium carrots peeled and chopped

2 stalks celery chopped

1 medium onion peeled and chopped

1 clove garlic peeled and minced

1 tsp dried mustard

½ tsp smoked paprika

¼ cup all-purpose flour

1 bottle lager beer or ale 12-ounce

4 cups chicken broth

½ cup heavy cream

2 cups shredded sharp cheddar cheese

1 cup shredded smoked Gouda cheese

Directions:

1. Press the Sauté button on the Instant Pot and melt butter. Add carrots, celery, and onion. Cook, stirring often, until softened, about 5 minutes. Add garlic and cook until fragrant, about 30 seconds, then add mustard and paprika and stir well.

2. Add flour and stir well to combine, then cook for 1 minute. Slowly stir in beer, scraping the bottom of pot well, then add broth. Press the Cancel button.

3. Close lid, set steam release to Sealing, press the Manual button, and set time to 5 minutes. When the timer beeps, let pressure release naturally, about 15 minutes. Open lid and purée mixture with an immersion blender. Stir in cream, then stir in cheese 1 cup

+ YOUR DESSERTS:

Cheesecake Mint Oreo

Time - 120 m | **Servings** - 10

Ingredients:

½ cup crushed graham cracker cookies

1 tbsp unsweetened cocoa powder

2 tbsp butter melted

12 oz cream cheese room temperature

½ cup sugar

¼ cup heavy cream

¼ cup sour cream

1 tsp vanilla extract

⅛ tsp mint extract

3-4 drops green food coloring (or more to achieve desired color optional)

1 tbsp all-purpose flour

2 eggs room temperature

1 egg yolk room temperature

8 whole Oreo cookies coarsely chopped, regular or mint flavored

1 cup Water

To Finish:

1 cup whipped cream or whipped topping

8 whole Oreo cookies coarsely chopped, regular or mint flavored

Chocolate sauce for garnish

Directions:

1. Coat the inside of a 7 inch springform pan with nonstick spray, then line bottom and sides with parchment paper.

2. In a small bowl, combine graham cracker crumbs, cocoa powder and melted butter until uniform. Press evenly into the bottom of the springform pan (use the bottom of a measuring cup as a press). Place in the freezer for 10 minutes.

3. Meanwhile, in a medium bowl, use a hand mixer to beat cream cheese and sugar for one minute. Add cream, sour cream, vanilla, mint extract, food coloring and flour and beat for one minute.

4. Add all eggs and beat just until combined. Do not overmix. Fold in chopped Oreo cookies.

5. Pour batter evenly into pan. Tap the pan on the counter several times to force any bubbles to the surface. Pop bubbles with a toothpick or fork.

6. Pour one cup of water in the Instant Pot and insert the steam rack. Carefully lower the springform pan on to the steam rack.

7. Using the display panel select the MANUAL or PRESSURE COOK function. Use the +/- keys and program the Instant Pot for 35 minutes.

8. When the time is up, let the pressure naturally release for 10 minutes, then quick-release the remaining pressure.

9. Carefully remove the pan from the pot to a wire rack. Use a paper towel to soak up any water on top of the cheesecake.

10. Allow to cool to room temperature, then remove the sides of the springform. Parchment will have wrinkled during cooking. Peel it back and re-wrap it around the cheesecake, smoothing the sides as you go. Cover and refrigerate at least 4 hours or overnight.

11. Unwrap the cheesecake, remove pan bottom and parchment. Place cheesecake on a serving plate.

12. Before serving, top with whipped cream, chopped Oreo cookies and a drizzle of chocolate sauce.

THANK YOU, YOU'RE DOING FINE!

○ *DAY: 14*

<u>RECOMMENDATION:</u>

14.Fresh plant foods must be present in the daily diet. They contain fiber, which is very helpful in removing bile from the gallbladder.

1. YOUR BREAKFAST:

Peach Melba Steel-Cut Oats

Time - 20 m | **Servings** - 6

Ingredients:

1 ½ cups steel cut oats

5 cups Water

½ cup pure maple syrup

pinch salt

2 cups peaches sliced, fresh or frozen

1 cup raspberries fresh or frozen

¼ cup chia seeds

Frozen Whipped Cream Dollops

Directions:

1. Add oats, water, syrup, salt, and peaches to the pressure cooker pot and stir.

2. Secure the lid and turn pressure release knob to a sealed position. Cook at high pressure for 10 minutes.

3. When cooking is complete, use a natural release for 10 minutes (can also use a full natural release, if not in a hurry). If liquid sprays through valve, turn back to the sealed position and allow to cool for 5-10 more minutes.

4. Sprinkle chia seeds over the top and stir in quickly, so they don't clump together. Scatter the raspberries over the top and

place the lid back on for 10 minutes to allow chia seeds to swell and raspberries to release some of their juices.

5. Serve hot with a frozen whipped cream dollop in the center.

2. YOUR LUNCH:

Creamy Broccoli Soup

Time - 20 m | **Servings** - 5

Ingredients:

1 cup red onion diced

2 cloves garlic minced

½ cup carrot diced

2 medium heads Broccoli about 3 cups of chopped stems and about 3 cups florets cut into small pieces

1 teaspoon salt

1 teaspoon thyme dried

2 ½ cups Water

15 ounce white beans rinsed and drained thoroughly (1 can)

1 tablespoon nutritional yeast optional

¼ cup parsley chopped

A few turns black peppercorns

Directions:

1. Press the sauté button on the Instant Pot, allow it to heat up for 2 minutes and then add the onion, garlic, carrot, broccoli (stems and florets), salt and thyme. Cook for 3 minutes, stirring frequently so nothing sticks to the bottom of the pot.

2. Turn off the Instant Pot, add the water and stir. Lock the lid into place, making sure the nozzle is in the sealing position.

3. Use the manual mode and set the timer for 4 minutes. When the timer goes off, use the quick release method.

4. When the pressure is totally down, take off the lid and remove about half of the broccoli florets and place them in a bowl. You don't have to take your time with this. Use a slotted

spoon and just fish a few spoonfuls out. No biggie if you pick up other veggies with your spoon along the way.

5. Now add the white beans and the nutritional yeast (if using) to the Instant Pot and allow to cool for about 10 minutes. Stirring the soup will help it cool faster.

6. When it's cool, blend the soup (minus the broccoli florets that you just reserved) in batches in your blender (or all in one go with a blender stick), until all of the soup is creamy and smooth.

7. When all of the soup is blended, add the reserved broccoli florets back into the pot, along with the parsley, black pepper and a little more salt to taste (if needed). Stir and let cool completely before you place in a container and store in the fridge.

3. YOUR SALAD:

Carrot Salad

Time - 20 m | **Servings** - 6

Ingredients:

½ tsp ground cumin

½ tsp ground coriander

½ tsp sweet paprika

water

Kosher salt

2 lb carrots, peeled and cut into medallions

1 celery stalk, chopped

¾ tsp harissa spice

1 to 2 garlic cloves, minced

1 celery stick finely chopped

½ cup chopped fresh cilantro (mint or parsley would work as well)

1 to 2 tbsp fresh lemon juice

3 tbsp Extra virgin olive oil (I used Early Harvest Greek extra virgin olive oil)

3 tbsp toasted sesame seeds, optional

Directions:

1. Bring a large pot of salted water to a boil. Add carrots and cook for about 20 minutes until nice and tender. Drain.

2. Transfer the cooked carrots immediately to a large mixing bowl. And while nice and warm, season with a dash kosher salt, and the spices (harissa spice, cumin, coriander and paprika). Add minced garlic, celery, cilantro, lemon juice and extra virgin olive oil.

3. If you like, add a sprinkle of toasted sesame seeds. Give the carrot salad a good toss to combine. Set the carrot salad aside for a bit before serving (it's best served at room temperature).

4. YOUR DINNER:

Beef Stroganoff

Time - 60 m | **Servings** - 6

Ingredients:

1 large onion diced (about 1 cup)

1 ¼ lbs boneless beef sirloin steak cut into thin strips

1 tsp paprika

½ tsp garlic powder

4 cups uncooked extra-wide egg noodles

2 cups water

2 tsp Worcestershire sauce

1 can Condensed Cream 10 ½ ounces

¼ cup sour cream

2 tbsp chopped fresh parsley

Directions:

1. Season the beef with salt and pepper. Layer the onion, beef, paprika, garlic powder and noodles in a 6 quart Instant Pot. Pour the broth and Worcestershire over the noodles and spoon the soup on top (the order is important, so don't stir until after the cooking is done).

2. Lock the lid and close the pressure release valve. Pressure cook on High pressure, setting the timer to 8 minutes (timer will begin counting down once pressure is reached- it takes about 15 minutes). When done, press Cancel and use the quick release method to release the pressure.

3. Stir in the sour cream and let stand for 5 minutes uncovered. Season to taste and sprinkle with the parsley before serving.

+ YOUR DESSERTS:

Strawberry Jam

Time - 60 m | **Servings** - 5

Ingredients:

4 cups quartered fresh strawberries

2 ½ cups sugar

¼ cup lemon juice

Directions:

1. Combine strawberries, sugar, and lemon juice in the Instant Pot. Select SAUTÉ and adjust to NORMAL. Bring mixture to a full boil for about 8 minutes, stirring frequently. Press CANCEL. Secure the lid on the pot. Close the pressure-release valve.

2. Select MANUAL and cook at high pressure for 8 minutes. When cooking is complete, use a natural release to depressurize. Press CANCEL. Remove the lid. Mash berries with a potato masher. Select SAUTÉ and adjust to NORMAL. Bring mixture to a full boil. Boil for 5 minutes or until mixture reaches gel stage (220°F) stirring frequently. Press CANCEL.

3. Ladle into half-pint glass jars. Seal jars. Store up to 3 weeks in the refrigerator.

THANK YOU, YOU'RE DOING FINE!

III. *BLUE* WEEK

15 16 17 18 19 20 21

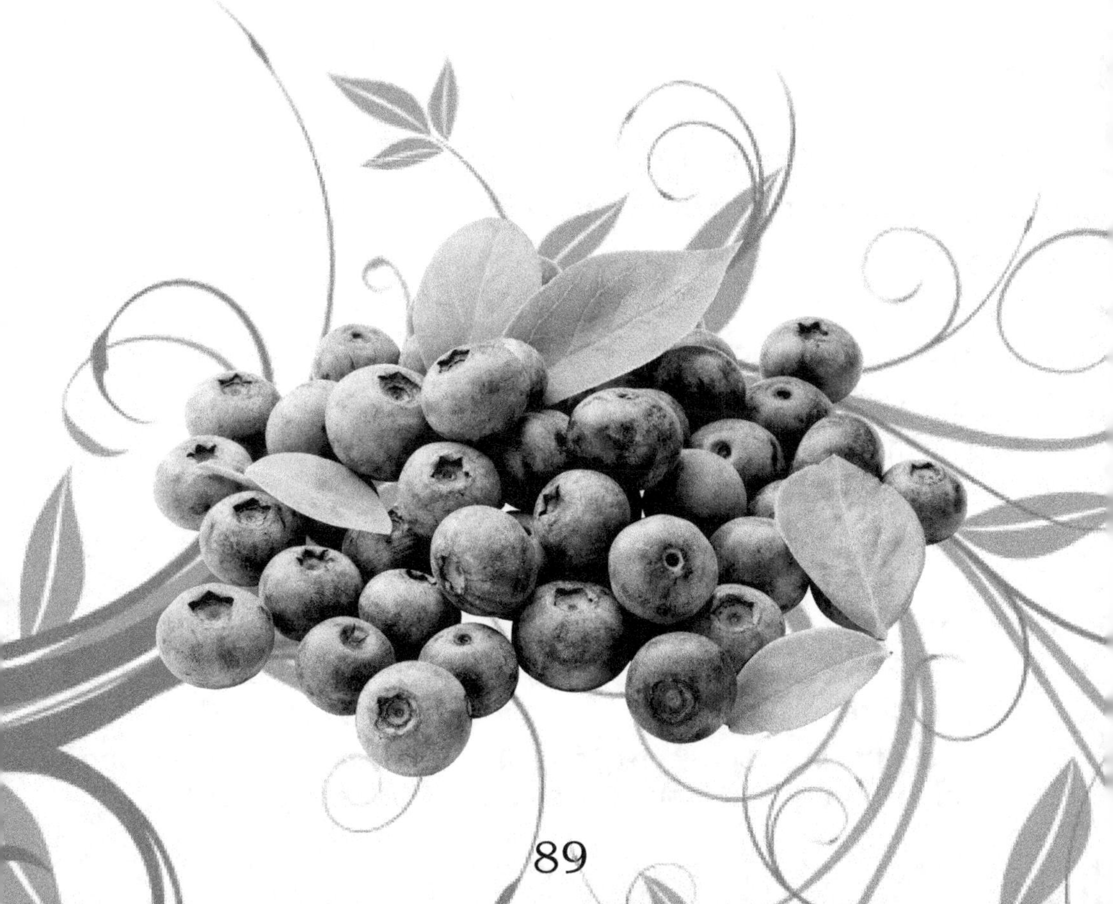

○ *DAY: 15*

RECOMMENDATION:

15.Most people hear about calories in foods, as well as proteins, fats and carbohydrates. Yes, these are important elements, but there are equally important ones - vitamins and minerals in food. And only initial products contain them. Cooked foods, such as baked goods, have fewer vitamins and minerals than their original foods, grains. Eat primary sources of food, and also drink vitamin and mineral supplements and omega-3 for prevention.

1. YOUR BREAKFAST:

Peach French Toast Casserole

Time - 40 m | **Servings** - 4

Ingredients:

4 tsp unsalted butter divided

6 slices whole grain bread cut into ½-inch cubes (about 4 cups)

2 large eggs

1 cup whole milk

½ tsp ground cinnamon

¾ cup packed-in-juice canned peaches

2 tbsp pecans chopped

1 tsp confectioners' sugar

4 tbsp maple syrup

Directions:

1. Place the steam rack in the inner pot and add 1 cup water to the bottom of the pot.
2. Coat the interior of a 1-quart (1l) soufflé dish with 1 teaspoon of the butter and then add the bread cubes to the dish.

3. In a medium bowl, combine the eggs, milk, and cinnamon. Whisk to combine, and then add the peaches and canning juice. Stir to combine.

4. Pour the egg mixture over the bread cubes and gently press the cubes into egg mixture until thoroughly coated in the mixture.

5. Cut the remaining butter into small pieces and evenly distribute over top of the bread cubes. Loosely cover the soufflé dish with aluminum foil.

6. Cover, lock the lid, and flip the steam release handle to the sealing position. Select Pressure Cook (Low) and set the cook time for 30 minutes. When the cook time is complete, quick release the pressure.

7. Open the lid. Carefully transfer the dish to a cooling rack and let the casserole cool for 10 minutes.

8. Garnish with the pecans and dust with the confectioners' sugar. Cut into 4 equal-sized portions and then drizzle 1 tablespoon maple syrup over top of each portion just before serving. Serve warm.

<u>2. YOUR LUNCH:</u>

Minestrone Soup

Time - 20 m | **Servings** - 5

Ingredients:

½ cup yellow onion chopped

2 cloves garlic minced

½ cup Zucchini chopped

½ red bell pepper diced (about ½ cup)

1 cup green beans fresh, string removed and cut into thirds

1 cup Eggplant cut into cubes

1 stalk celery diced

½ cup carrot chopped

1 small russet potato diced

¼ cup parsley chopped

15.5 ounce garbanzo beans rinsed and drained well, 1 can.

12 ounce tomatoes diced, 1 can

2 teaspoons basil dried

2 teaspoons oregano

10 turns black pepper

1 teaspoon salt

3 cups Water

Directions:

1. Prep and measure out all of the ingredients first. This will make it super easy to throw together.

2. Press Sauté on your Instant Pot and let the inner pot heat up for 2 minutes.

3. Add all of the ingredients, except for the water and sauté for 5 minutes, stirring regularly so that nothing sticks to the bottom of the pot (onion, garlic, zucchini, bell pepper, green beans, eggplant, celery, potato, parsley, garbanzo beans, tomatoes, basil, oregano, black pepper and salt). Add just a splash of water if the veggies start to stick.

4. Turn off the Instant Pot, add the water and stir. Lock the lid into place, making sure the nozzle is in the sealing position.

5. Use the Manual setting and set the timer for 10 minutes. When time is up, use the natural release method. When all of the pressure is out of the Instant Pot, take off the lid and allow to cool.

3. YOUR SALAD:

Roasted Vegetables & Barley

Time - 60 m | **Servings** - 5

Ingredients:

2 tsp/ 3.9 g harissa spice, divided

¾ tsp/ 1.95 g smoked paprika, divided

Early Harvest Greek extra virgin olive oil

2 scallions (green onions), trimmed and chopped (both whites and greens)

1 garlic clove, minced

2 oz / 56 g chopped fresh parsley

2 tbsp/30 ml fresh squeezed lemon juice

1 cup/163 g dry pearl barley, washed

water

2 whole zucchini squash, diced

1 red bell pepper, cored, diced

1 yellow bell pepper, cored, diced

1 medium red onion, diced

salt and pepper

Feta cheese, to taste (optional)

Toasted pine nuts, to taste (optional)

Directions:

1. Preheat oven to 425 degrees F.

2. Place pearl barley and 2 ½ cups (591 ml) water in a saucepan. Bring to a boil, then turn heat down to low. Cover and cook for 40 to 45 minutes or until the barley is cooked through (should be tender but maintains some chew).

3. While barley is cooking, place diced vegetables (zucchini, bell peppers, and red onion) on a large baking sheet. Season with salt, pepper, 1 ½ tsp harissa spice, and ½ tsp smoked paprika. Drizzle with extra virgin olive oil. Toss to coat. Spread evenly in one layer on the baking sheet. Roast in heated oven for 25 minutes or so.

4. When barley is ready, drain any excess water. Season with salt, pepper, ½ tsp harissa spice and ¼ tsp smoked paprika. Toss to combine.

5. Transfer cooked barley to a large mixing bowl. Add roasted veggies. Add chopped scallions, garlic, and fresh parsley. Dress with lemon juice and a good drizzle of Early Harvest extra virgin olive oil. Toss. If you like, top with crumbled feta and toasted pine nuts.

6. Serve warm, at room temperature, or cold! Enjoy.

<u>4. YOUR DINNER:</u>

Tahini Lamb Meatballs with Couscous
Time - 120 m | **Servings** - 4

Ingredients:
Lamb Meatballs and Couscous Ingredients:
½ cup Tahini Sauce divided
3 tbsp panko bread crumbs
1 lb ground lamb
¼ cup chopped fresh mint divided
1 tsp ground cinnamon divided
1 tsp ground cumin divided
¾ tsp table salt divided
1 tbsp extra-virgin olive oil
1 onion chopped fine
⅛ tsp cayenne pepper
1 cup chicken broth plus extra as needed
1 cup couscous
½ cup jarred roasted red peppers rinsed, patted dry, and chopped
1 tbsp teaspoon grated lemon zest plus 1juice
⅓ cup Quick Pickled Onions
Tahini Sauce Ingredients:
½ cup tahini
½ cup Water
¼ cup lemon juice (2 lemons)
2 garlic cloves minced
Quick Pickled Onions Ingredients:
1 cup red wine vinegar
⅓ cup sugar
⅛ tsp table salt
1 red onion halved and sliced thin through root end

Directions:

Tahini Sauce Instructions

1. Whisk all Tahini sauce ingredients in bowl until smooth (mixture will appear broken at first). Season with salt and pepper to taste. Let sit at room temperature for at least 30 minutes to allow flavors to meld. (Sauce can be refrigerated for up to 4 days; bring to room temperature before serving.)

Quick Pickled Onions Instructions

2. Microwave vinegar, sugar, and salt in medium bowl until simmering, 1 to 2 minutes. Add onion and let sit, stirring occasionally, for 45 minutes. Drain onion and return to now-empty bowl. (Drained onions can be refrigerated for up to 1 week.)

Lamb Meatballs and Couscous

3. Using fork, mash ¼ cup Tahini Sauce and panko together in bowl to form paste. Add ground lamb, 2 tablespoons mint, ½ teaspoon cinnamon, ½ teaspoon cumin, and ½ teaspoon salt, and knead with hands until thoroughly combined. Pinch off and roll mixture into twelve 1 ½ inch meatballs.

4. Using highest Sauté function, heat oil in Instant Pot until shimmering. Add onion and remaining ¼ teaspoon salt and cook until onion is softened, about 5 minutes. Stir in remaining ½ teaspoon cinnamon, remaining ½ teaspoon cumin, and cayenne and cook until fragrant, about 30 seconds. Stir in broth, scraping up any browned bits. Add meatballs to pot. Lock lid in place and close pressure release valve. Select Pressure Cook function and cook for 1 minute.

5. Turn off Instant Pot and quick-release pressure. Carefully remove lid, allowing steam to escape away from you. Using slotted spoon, transfer meatballs to plate, tent with aluminum foil, and let rest while cooking couscous. (You should have about 2 cups cooking liquid remaining in pot; add extra broth as needed to equal 2 cups.)

6. Using highest Sauté function, bring liquid in pot to simmer. Stir in couscous, red peppers, and lemon zest and juice. Turn off Instant Pot, cover, and let sit for 10 minutes. Fluff couscous gently with fork and transfer to serving dish. Arrange meatballs on top and drizzle with remaining ¼

cup Tahini Sauce. Sprinkle with pickled onions and remaining 2 tablespoons mint. Serve.

+ YOUR DESSERTS:

Triple Citrus Cheesecake

Time - 6 h | **Servings** - 7

Ingredients:

1 ½ cups graham cracker or vanilla wafer crumbs

2 tablespoons sugar

4 tablespoons melted butter

16 ounces cream cheese, softened

½ cup sugar

1 tablespoon flour

¼ teaspoon salt

2 teaspoons vanilla

2 tablespoons orange juice

2 eggs

½ teaspoon freshly grated lime zest

2 cups water

Fresh orange segments (optional)

Directions:

1. Lightly spray a 6-or 7-inch springform pan with cooking spray. Cut a piece of parchment paper to fit the bottom of the pan. Place in the pan and spray again; set aside.

2. Combine crackers, the 2 tablespoons sugar, and butter in a bowl; mix well. Press into bottom and about 2 inches up the sides of the pan.

3. In a large bowl beat cream cheese, the ½ cup sugar, flour, salt, vanilla, and orange juice until smooth and creamy. Addeggs, beating just until combined. Stir in citrus zests. Pour into prepared crust.

4. Pour the water into the Instant Pot. Place the trivet in the bottom of the pot. Cut a piece of foil the same size as a paper

towel. Place the foil under the paper towel and place the pan on top of the paper towel. Wrap the bottom of the pan in the foil, with the paper towel as a barrier.

5. Fold an 18-inch-long piece of foil into thirds lengthwise. Place under the pan and use the two sides as a sling to place cheesecake in thepot. Secure the lid on the pot. Close the pressure-release valve.

6. Select manual and cook at high pressure for 35 minutes. When cooking is complete, use a natural pressure release to depressurize.

7. Remove the cheesecake from the pot using the sling. Cool on a wire rack for 1 hour and then refrigerate for at least 4 hours. Carefully remove pan sides. Top cheesecake with fresh orange segments if desired.

THANK YOU, YOU CAN DO EVERYTHING!

○ *DAY: 16*

<u>RECOMMENDATION:</u>

16.Everyone around is repeating that it is good to drink freshly squeezed juices. But eating whole fruits is much healthier. Do not drink juices every day, because there is high acidity, a lot of sugars, and in general nothing else. Drink them occasionally as a dessert.

<u>1. YOUR BREAKFAST:</u>

Blackberry Soy Milk Yogurt

Time - 14 h | **Servings** - 4

Ingredients:

4 cups plain, sweetened soy milk

3 tbsp plain, dairy-free yogurt (soy, cashew, or almond)

2 tsp vanilla extract

1 pint fresh blackberries

2 tbsp pistachios roughly chopped

4 tbsp honey

Directions:

1. Add the soy milk and yogurt to the inner pot. Stir well.

2. Cover and lock the lid, but leave the steam release handle in the venting position. Select Yogurt and set the cook time for 14 hours. When the cook time is complete, remove the lid and stir in the vanilla extract.

3. Allow the yogurt to cool slightly, and then transfer to a large, seal-able glass jar, and seal tightly. Place in the refrigerator to chill and thicken for a minimum of 4 hours.

4. To serve, transfer the chilled yogurt to serving bowls. Top each serving with ½ cup blackberries and 1-½ teaspoons

pistachios, and then drizzle 1 tablespoon honey over top. Store in the refrigerator for up to 5 days.

2. YOUR LUNCH:

Best Minestrone Soup

Time - 10 m | **Servings** - 8

Ingredients:

2 tablespoons olive oil

1 medium onion chopped, about 1 ¼ cups

3 tablespoon tablespoons parsley minced fresh, or 1 dried parsley

1 clove garlic minced

43.5 ounces chicken broth fat-free, lower-sodium, 3 cans

16 ounce pinto beans undrained, 1 can

4 medium tomatoes peeled and coarsely chopped, about 4 cups

2 stalks celery sliced, about 1 cup

2 medium carrots sliced, about 1 cup

1 medium Zucchini halved lengthwise and sliced, about 2 cups

½ cup elbow macaroni uncooked

2 teaspoons basil dried, crushed

½ teaspoon salt

½ teaspoon Italian seasoning dried

⅛ teaspoon red pepper dried crushed

5 cups kale leaves packed, coarsely chopped and stemmed

Parmesan cheese Freshly grated

Directions:

1. Remove lid from a 6-quart Instant Pot. Press [Sauté]. Use [Adjust] to select "Normal" mode. When the word "Hot" appears, swirl in oil.

2. Add onion. Cook, stirring frequently, 5 minutes or until onion is tender but not brown. Add parsley and garlic. Cook, stirring constantly for 30 seconds. Immediately add chicken broth and beans.

3. Stir in tomato, celery, carrots, zucchini, elbow macaronis, basil, Italian seasoning, and crushed red pepper . Turn cooker off. Close and lock the lid of the Instant Pot.

4. Turn the steam release handle to "Sealing" position. Press [Manual]; select "High Pressure," and use [-] or [+] to choose 6 minutes pressure cooking time. When time is up, turn cooker off. Open the cooker using Quick Pressure Release. Press [Sauté]. Use [Adjust] to select "More" mode.

5. Add kale, stirring frequently, 2 to 3 minutes or until soup just comes to a boil and kale wilts. Turn cooker off.

6. Ladle soup into bowls; sprinkle with Parmesan cheese.

3. YOUR SALAD:

Quick Organic

Time - 20 m | **Servings** - 6

Ingredients:

1 head raw cauliflower, cut into florets

1 whole bunch parsley, stems partially removed

3 to 4 Roma tomatoes, very small diced or chopped

1 English cucumber (hot house cucumber), chopped

½ red onion, finely chopped

1 to 2 garlic cloves, minced

Kosher salt and pepper

Juice of 2 lemons

Extra virgin olive oil

Directions:

1. Place the cauliflower florets in the bowl of a food processor fitted with a blade. Pulse a few times until the cauliflower turns rice-like in texture.

2. Transfer the finely chopped cauliflower into a larger bowl. Add the parsley, tomatoes, cucumbers, and onions. Give the salad a quick toss to combine.

3. Now, add minced garlic and season with salt and pepper. Finish with fresh lemon juice and a good drizzle of extra virgin olive oil (about 2 tbsp). Give the salad one more good toss to combine.

4. For best results, set the cauliflower salad aside for a few minutes before serving to allow the cauliflower to soften and absorb some of the dressing. You can also cover and chill for later. Enjoy!

4. YOUR DINNER:

Rigatoni & Tomatoes and Pancetta

Time - 60 m | **Servings** - 6

Ingredients:

4 oz pancetta chopped fine

1 onion chopped fine

¼ tsp table salt

3 garlic cloves minced

2 anchovy fillets rinsed, patted dry, and minced

2 tsp fennel seeds lightly cracked

¼ tsp red pepper flakes

1 can diced tomatoes 28 ounce

2 cups chicken broth

1 ½ cups Water

1 lb rigatoni

¼ cup grated Pecorino Romano cheese plus extra for serving

2 tbsp minced fresh parsley

Directions:

1. Using highest sauté function, cook pancetta in Instant Pot, stirring often, until browned and fat is well rendered, 6 to 10 minutes. Using slotted spoon, transfer pancetta to paper towel–lined plate; set aside for serving.

2. Add onion and salt to fat left in pot and cook, using highest sauté function, until onion is softened, about 5 minutes. Stir in

garlic, anchovies, fennel seeds, and pepper flakes and cook until fragrant, about 1 minute. Stir in tomatoes and their juice, broth, and water, scraping up any browned bits, then stir in pasta.

3. Lock lid in place and close pressure release valve. Select Pressure Cook function on High and cook for 5 minutes. Turn off Instant Pot and quick-release pressure. Carefully remove lid, allowing steam to escape away from you.

4. Stir in Pecorino and season with salt and pepper to taste. Transfer to serving dish and let sit until sauce thickens slightly, about 5 minutes. Sprinkle with parsley and reserved pancetta. Serve, passing extra Pecorino separately.

+ YOUR DESSERTS:

Chocolate-Bourbon Lava Cakes

Time - 30 m | **Servings** - 10

Ingredients:

1 stick (4 ounces) unsalted butter, plus more for the ramekins

6 ounces bittersweet (65% to 74% cacao) chocolate, chopped (or use chips)

¾ cup confectioners' sugar

⅛ teaspoon fine sea salt

3 large eggs, plus 1 egg yolk

1 tablespoon bourbon or vanilla extract

6 tablespoons all-purpose flour

Flaky sea salt, for serving

Crème fraîche, sour cream, or ice cream, for serving

Directions:

1. In a microwave safe medium bowl, melt the butter with the chocolate (or do this in a small saucepan over low heat). Meanwhile, butter four 6-ounce ramekins.

2. To the bowl with the butter/chocolate mixture, add the confectioners' sugar and salt and whisk until cool to the

touch. Whisk in the whole eggs and egg yolk, followed by the bourbon and flour. Distribute the mixture evenly among the four ramekins. Cover each with aluminum foil.

3. Pour 1 cup water into the pressure cooker pot. Place a steamer rack/trivet at the bottom of the pot. Stack the ramekins on the rack. You should be able to fit three on the bottom with the fourth placed on top in the center.

4. Lock the lid into place and cook on high pressure for 9 minutes. Manually release the pressure.

5. With tongs, remove the ramekins from the pot and allow them to sit for 3 minutes, still covered with foil. Then remove the foil and run a knife around the edge of each cake. Flip each cake onto a serving plate. Sprinkle with sea salt and top with crème fraîche or ice cream, if you like. Serve immediately.

THANK YOU, YOU CAN DO EVERYTHING!

○ *DAY: 17*

<u>RECOMMENDATION:</u>

17.If you live in a multi-storey residential building, then walk instead of taking the elevator. If you have a lot of 10 or more floors, start with at least 2-3.

1. YOUR BREAKFAST:

Breakfast Burrito Bowl

Time - 20 m | **Servings** - 4

Ingredients:

6 eggs

3 tbsp melted butter

1 tsp salt

¼ tsp pepper

½ pound cooked breakfast sausage

½ cup shredded sharp cheddar cheese

½ cup salsa

½ cup sour cream

1 avocado cubed

¼ cup green onion diced

Directions:

1. In large bowl, mix eggs, melted butter, salt, and pepper. Press the Sauté button and then press the Adjust button to set the heat to Less.

2. Add eggs to Instant Pot. and cook for 5–7 minutes while gently moving with rubber spatula. When eggs begin to firm up, add cooked breakfast sausage and cheese and continue to cook until eggs are fully cooked. Press the Cancel button.

3. Divide eggs into four bowls and top with salsa, sour cream, avocado, and green onion.

2. YOUR LUNCH:

Poblano Corn Chowder

Time - 150 m | **Servings** - 8

Ingredients:

1 tablespoon olive oil

1 large onion diced

2 large carrots peeled and diced

2 stalks celery peeled and diced

1 lagre poblano pepper ribs and seeds removed, finely diced*

2 cloves garlic minced

3 ½ cups chicken broth

½ teaspoon thyme dried

1 teaspoon salt

½ teaspoon black pepper

dash red pepper flakes

4 cups potatoes peeled and cubed

3 tablespoons cornstarch

3 tablespoons Water

2 cups half and half

4 cups corn frozen

Directions:

1. Select Saute and add oil to the Instant Pot. When oil is hot, add the onion, carrots, and celery, and cook, stirring occasionally, until tender, about 5 minutes.

2. Add poblano pepper and garlic. Cook for 1 more minute.

3. Add half of the chicken broth, thyme, salt, pepper, red pepper flakes, and parsley to the pot.

4. Put the steamer basket in the pressure cooker pot. Add the diced potatoes.

5. Lock the lid in place, select Manual and adjust to high pressure cooking. Set time to cook for 4 minutes. When timer beeps, turn off pressure cooker, allow natural release for 5 minutes, then do a quick pressure release. Carefully remove potatoes and steamer basket from the pressure cooking pot.

6. In a small bowl, dissolve cornstarch in 3 tablespoons water. Select Simmer and add cornstarch mixture to the pot stirring constantly until mixture thickens.

7. Gradually whisk in the remaining chicken broth. Stir in half and half, corn, and potatoes; heat through but do not bring to a boil.

8. Add a dash of hot sauce, if desired. Garnish with fresh parsley. Enjoy!

3. YOUR SALAD:

Szechuan Pea

Time - 30 m | **Servings** - 4

Ingredients:

1 avocado, cubed (1 cup)

2 Tbs. lemon juice

¼ cup olive oil

3 Tbs. red wine vinegar

1 Tbs. vegan Szechuan sauce

2 tsp. sugar

2 14-oz. cans black-eyed peas, rinsed and drained

1 medium green bell pepper, chopped (1 cup)

½ cup chopped red onion

1 jalapeno chile, seeded and finely minced (2 Tbs).

1 clove garlic, minced (1 tsp).

Directions:

1. Toss together black-eyed peas, bell pepper, onion, jalapeño, and garlic in large bowl. Toss avocado with lemon juice in separate bowl. Add avocado to black-eyed pea mixture.

2. Whisk together oil, vinegar, Szechuan sauce, and sugar in bowl used for avocado. Add black-eyed pea mixture, and toss to mix.

4. YOUR DINNER:

Lemon-Herb Chicken

Time - 60 m | **Servings** - 4

Ingredients:

1 Tbsp. oil

1 ½ lbs boneless, skinless chicken breasts cut into strips

½ cup Water

1 jar INSTANT POT Zesty Lemon Herb Sauce 15 oz

Directions:

1. HEAT oil in Instant Pot using SAUTÉ setting on high heat. Add chicken; cook 5 min., stirring frequently.

2. ADD water and sauce. Do not stir. Close and lock lid. Turn Pressure Release Valve to Sealing position.

3. COOK 6 min. using HIGH PRESSURE COOK/ MANUAL setting. When timer goes off, use Quick Pressure Release to release pressure before carefully opening lid.

+ YOUR DESSERTS:

Jalapeño Cheddar Cornbread

Time - 60 m | **Servings** - 7

Ingredients:

1 cup yellow cornmeal

¾ cup all-purpose flour

2 teaspoons baking powder

2-3 jalapeño peppers seeded and finely chopped, divided

1.25 cups sharp cheddar cheese grated, divided

1 cup fresh or frozen corn

¼ cup green scallions thinly sliced (optional)

¾ cup buttermilk or ¾ cup milk with 1 tsp of lemon juice

¼ cup butter, melted

¼ cup honey

2 eggs, cold

1 teaspoon salt

Directions:

1. Add 1 cup of water to the Instant Pot. Grease and lightly coat 7" cake pan with corn meal and set aside.
2. In a large mixing bowl, combine the cornmeal, flour, baking powder and salt. Mix well.
3. Add the grated cheese, chopped jalapeño and scallions (save 1 tablespoon of each to garnish)
4. Add the corn kernels to the flour mixture. Mix gently until well coated.
5. In a separate bowl, whisk together the buttermilk, melted butter, honey, and eggs.
6. Pour over mixed dry ingredients and stir gently with a spoon until just combined.
7. Pour into the prepared pan and garnish with the remaining jalapeño and grated cheese.
8. Cover the cake pan with paper towel and aluminum foil. Place the cake pan on the trivet and gently put the trivet in the Instant Pot insert.
9. Cook on Manual(Hi) for 25 minutes with NPR. You can optionally broil for 2 minutes to get browned cheese on top. We enjoy the bread as is!
10. Enjoy warm.

THANK YOU, YOU CAN DO EVERYTHING!

○ *DAY: 18*

RECOMMENDATION:

18.If you think you need to eat less to lose weight, this is not necessarily the case. The concentration of nutrients on the volume of food is important. Example: for energy value, 1 bar of chocolate = approximately 2.5 pounds of vegetable salad! Therefore, to reduce body fat, it is important to replace energetically dense foods with energetically less dense ones. Then you will gorge on and lose weight at the same time. Eat more vegetables, preferably fresh (salads or whole).

1. YOUR BREAKFAST:

Sausage and Kale Egg Muffins

Time - 15 m | **Servings** - 2

Ingredients:

1 tsp avocado oil

2 tsp bacon fat (or more avocado oil)

4 ounces fully cooked chicken sausage diced

4 small kale leaves any variety, finely chopped

½ tsp kosher salt

½ tsp ground black pepper

4 large eggs

¼ cup heavy (whipping) cream or full-fat coconut milk

4 tbsp shredded white cheddar or swiss cheese optional

1 cup Water

Directions:

1. Use the 1 teaspoon avocado oil to grease the bottom and insides of four silicone muffin cups (preferred), ceramic

ramekins, or half-pint mason jars. If you have a silicone egg bites mold, you can also use that for this recipe.

2. Set the Instant Pot to Sauté and melt the bacon fat. Add the sausage and sauté for 2 minutes. Add the chopped kale and ¼ teaspoon each of the salt and pepper. Sauté until the kale is wilted, 2 to 3 minutes longer.

3. Meanwhile, in a medium bowl, lightly beat together the eggs, cream, and remaining ¼ teaspoon each salt and pepper

4. Press Cancel. Divide the kale-sausage mixture among the four muffin cups. Pour the egg mixture evenly over the kale and sausage and stir lightly with a fork. If desired, top each with 1 tablespoon shredded cheese. Loosely cover the cups with foil or silicone lids.

5. Pour the water into the Instant Pot. Place the metal steam rack/trivet inside. Place the four muffin cups on top.

6. Secure the lid and set the steam release valve to Sealing. Press the Pressure Cook or Manual button and set the cook time to 5 minutes.

7. When the Instant Pot beeps, allow the pressure to release naturally for 10 minutes, then carefully switch the steam release valve to Venting.

8. Carefully remove the muffins from the Instant Pot. Serve hot or warm.

2. YOUR LUNCH:

Pho Ga

Time - 60 m | **Servings** - 5

Ingredients:

1 tbsp canola oil

½ red onion peeled and cut in half

1 inch piece fresh ginger root & 1 clove garlic

2 tsp coriander seeds & 1 cinnamon stick

2 whole star anise

2 lbs bone-in, skin-on chicken thighs (about 4 chicken thighs)

1 tbsp fish sauce

8 cups Water

12 ounces rice noodles

1 cup fresh cilantro leaves stems removed

1 cup bean sprouts

1 Jalapeno pepper stem removed and thinly sliced

Directions:

1. Select Sauté and add the canola oil to the inner pot. Heat the oil until it shimmers, and then add the onion. Sauté for 2–3 minutes, or until the onion is lightly browned and slightly translucent. Add the ginger root, garlic, coriander seeds, cinnamon stick, and star anise.

2. Sauté for 1 additional minute, and then add the chicken thighs, fish sauce, and water.

3. Cover, lock the lid, and flip the steam release handle to the sealing position. Select Pressure Cook (High) and set the cook time for 20 minutes. When the cook time is complete, allow the pressure to release naturally (about 30 minutes).

4. While the broth is cooking, fill a large bowl with warm water and place the rice noodles in the bowl to soften (about 20 minutes).

5. Once the cooking time for the broth is complete, remove the lid and transfer the chicken thighs to a plate to cool slightly. When the thighs are cool enough, remove and discard the skin, shred, and discard the bones.

6. Drain the noodles. Place a fine mesh sieve over a large bowl, carefully remove the inner pot from the base, and strain the broth. Discard the solids and return the strained broth to the inner pot. Select Sauté and bring the broth to a simmer. Add the noodles and simmer for an additional 2–3 minutes. Add the chicken to the pot.

7. Using tongs, transfer the noodles to serving bowls, and then ladle in the broth and chicken. Top each serving with the cilantro leaves, bean sprouts, jalapeño slices, and a dollop of the Sriracha, if using.

<u>3. YOUR SALAD:</u>

Tuna with a Dijon Mustard

Time - 15 m | **Servings** - 7

Ingredients:

For the Tuna Salad

3 cans tuna, 5 ounces each (use quality tuna of your choice)

2 ½ celery stalks, chopped

½ English cucumber, chopped

4–5 whole small radishes, stems removed, chopped

3 green onions, both white and green parts, chopped

½ medium-sized red onion, finely chopped

½ cup cup pitted Kalamata olives, halved

1 bunch of parsley, stems removed, chopped (about 1 cup chopped fresh parsley)

10–15 fresh mint leaves, stems removed, finely chopped (about ½ cup chopped fresh mint)

Six slices heirloom tomatoes for serving

Homemade Pita chips or pita pockets for serving

For the Zesty Dijon Mustard Dressing

2 ½ tsp good quality Dijon mustard

Zest of 1 lime

1 ½ limes, juice of

⅓ cup Early Harvest extra virgin olive oil

½ tsp sumac

Pinch of salt and pepper

½ tsp crushed red pepper flakes, optional

Directions:

1. To make the zesty mustard vinaigrette, in a small bowl, whisk together the Dijon mustard, lime zest, and lime juice. Add the olive oil, sumac, salt and pepper, and crushed pepper flakes (if using), and whisk again until well-blended. Set aside briefly.

2. To make the tuna salad, in a large salad bowl, combine the tuna with the chopped vegetables, Kalamata olives, chopped fresh parsley and mint leaves. Mix gently with a wooden spoon.

3. Pour the dressing over the tuna salad. Mix again to make sure the tuna salad is evenly coated with the dressing. Cover and refrigerate for half an hour before serving. When ready to serve, toss the salad gently to refresh.

4. Serve in pita pockets for a sandwich dinner. Or to serve as an appetizer, transfer to a serving platter and add pita chips and sliced heirloom tomatoes on the side. If you like, serve a portion of the tuna salad over the sliced heirloom tomatoes. Enjoy!

4. YOUR DINNER:

BBQ Meatballs

Time - 60 m | **Servings** - 6

Ingredients:

2 lbs lean ground beef

½ cup finely chopped onions

¼ cup finely chopped fresh parsley

1 tbsp minced Garlic

2 tsp LEA & PERRINS Worcestershire Sauce

1 tsp salt

½ tsp black pepper

2 eggs beaten

1 cup dry bread crumbs divided

1 jar INSTANT POT Southern BBQ Sauce divided, 15 oz

½ cup fat-free reduced-sodium beef broth

Directions:

1. 1 cup water to INSTANT POT. Place trivet in pot.

2. Mix first 8 ingredients in large bowl just until blended. Add half the bread crumbs and 2 tbsp barbecue sauce; mix lightly. Gently mix in remaining bread crumbs.

3. Shape meat mixture into 40 meatballs (½ inch- 1 inch)

4. Place half the meatballs in single layer on trivet; cover with second layer of meatballs. Close and lock lid. Turn Pressure Release Valve to Sealing position.

5. Cook 7 min using MANUAL/HIGH PRESSURE COOK setting. When timer goes off, use Natural Pressure Release for 5 min., then do a Quick Pressure Release to release any remaining steam. Remove lid.

6. Use tongs to transfer meatballs to serving bowl; cover to keep warm. Remove trivet from INSTANT POT. Discard meat juices from pot. Rinse liner, then return liner to pot.

7. Add beef broth and remaining barbecue sauce to pot; stir. Cook using SAUTÉ setting 3 min. or until heated through, stirring frequently. Pour over meatballs; stir to evenly coat meatballs with sauce.

+ YOUR DESSERTS:

Coconut Flan

Time - 30 m | **Servings** - 6

Ingredients:

13.5 ounces Coconut Milk

12 ounces Evaporated Milk

14 ounces Condensed Milk

1 cup Sugar

1 cup Milk(full fat or 2%)

3 Eggs

1 pinch Salt

½ cup Desiccated Coconut

2 splashes Vanilla Extract

6" Aluminum cake tin/ flan mold

Fine mesh strainer

Directions:

1. To prepare the Caramel Syrup-In a saucepan/ the same aluminum cake tin, over medium heat, add the sugar and allow it to melt and reach a medium amber color syrup consistency. Make sure you don't stir in between and babysit this process for 5 mins)

2. Once the caramel is done, remove from heat(to prevent burning) and swirl the cake tin to fully cover the bottom.

3. Now pour all the other liquid ingredients, vanilla and coconut extracts, salt, and eggs in a blender and blend until well combined.

4. Pour the mixture through the mesh strainer into the prepared cake tin and cover using a foil.

5. Add 2 cups water into the IP inner pot and place the trivet.

6. Now use a foil sling to lower the cake tin onto the trivet inside the IP. Keep the foil strips folded down to prevent contact with the lid.

7. Cover the IP with the lid and turn the steam handle to sealing position and set the pressure cook mode for 15 mins on high pressure.

8. Open the IP lid using Natural Pressure Release.Carefully take out the flan tin and check the doneness. If the flan is cooked through, let it cool to room temp and then refrigerate for a minimum of 4 hours.(If the flan is not fully cooked, keep for another 1 min on high pressure and open using NPR) Tastes better when chilled overnight!

9. To unmold the flan, turn the flan tin upside down and set it on top of the serving plate and hold the plate and flan tin firmly together and then shake it firmly. Now gently lift the tin and there you have your fabulous dessert! Best had when chilled overnight.

10. Serve the flan cold, drizzled with some caramel syrup and shredded coconut sprinkled on top.

11. Tip Substitute coconut milk in this recipe with mango puree to create a Mango Flan.

THANK YOU, YOU CAN DO EVERYTHING!

○ *DAY: 19*

RECOMMENDATION:

19.Headaches are also associated with low mobility of the neck, as a result, less blood enters the brain than it should normally receive. Perform neck exercises for at least 5 days and this will already give a good result. Make smooth turns in different directions, turn your head.

1. YOUR BREAKFAST:

Tasty & Quickly

Time - 20 m | **Servings** - 4

Ingredients:

1 cup steel cut oats not quick cooking type

¼ cup brown sugar

2 tablespoons butter

pinch salt to taste

3 cups Water

½ cup dried cranberries for topping

½ cup slivered almonds for topping

Directions:

1. Put Oats, Brown Sugar, Butter, Salt, and Water into Instant Pot. Stir.

2. Close lid and make sure the vent is set to "sealing." Press the Manual or Pressure Cook button and adjust the timer to 12 minutes. Instant Pot will pressurize then the countdown timer will begin.

3. After the timer reaches zero, DO NOT release the steam valve yet. Let it "naturally release" it's pressure for 10-12 minutes. Then release the remaining steam by turning the pressure valve to "venting."

4. Once steam has escaped, remove the lid. Stir oatmeal until desired consistency then serve in individual bowls with dried cranberries and slivered almonds. (or whatever toppings you like). Clean up is a breeze! Enjoy!

2. YOUR LUNCH:

Tasty Beef Stew

Time - 40 m | **Servings** - 5

Ingredients:

1 ½ lbs Beef Stew Meat trimmed and cut into 1-2 inch chunks

1 tsp salt

1 tsp pepper

1 tsp Italian seasoning

1 tbsp olive oil

3 cloves garlic minced

1 medium onion finely chopped

3 carrots peeled and cut into slices

2 celery stalks chopped

2 ½ cups low-sodium beef broth or stock

2 tbsp Worcestershire sauce

10 oz tomato sauce 1 can

1 lb potatoes chopped into 1 inch chunks

2 tbsp cornstarch

Directions:

1. Season stew meat with salt, pepper and Italian seasoning
2. Add olive oil to the Instant Pot. Using the display panel select the SAUTE function.
3. When oil starts to sizzle, brown the meat on all sides. Meat will not be cooked through. Do not crowd the pot--you may have to work in batches. Transfer browned meat to a bowl, but leave as much liquid as possible in the pot.

4. Add garlic, onions, carrots and celery to the pot. Continue to sauté for 3-4 minutes (if it gets too dry, add additional 1 tbsp of olive oil)

5. Add beef broth to the pot and deglaze by using a wooden spoon to scrape the brown bits from the bottom of the pot.

6. Add beef back to the pot along with Worcestershire sauce, tomato sauce and potatoes.

7. Turn the pot off by selecting CANCEL, then secure the lid, making sure the vent is closed.

8. Using the display panel select the MANUAL function*. Use the +/- buttons and program the Instant Pot for 30 minutes.

9. When the time is up, let the pressure naturally release for 15 minutes, then quick-release the remaining pressure.

10. Mix together the cornstarch with 2 tbsp cold water in a small bowl and stir into the stew until thickened.

3. YOUR SALAD:

Roasted Eggplant Caprese

Time - 50 m | **Servings** - 5

Ingredients:

16 Oz. fresh mozzarella cheese, sliced

1 eggplant, sliced into ½-inch rounds

Salt

3 large or steak tomatoes, sliced into ½-inch rounds

Extra virgin olive oil

20 basil leaves, more for the dressing

Basil Vinaigrette (optional)

1 small garlic clove, chopped

1 cup packed basil leaves

¼ cup extra virgin olive oil

½ tbsp lime juice

Pinch crushed red pepper

Salt and pepper

Directions:

1. Preheat the oven to 425 degrees F.

2. Spread the eggplant slices on a large tray and sprinkle generously with salt. Leave for 30 minutes; the eggplant will "sweat out" it's bitterness. When ready, pat the eggplant dry.

3. Place the eggplant slices and the tomato slices on a large baking sheet. Drizzle with olive oil. Roast in the 425 F degree heated-oven for 10-15 minutes. Remove from the oven, but leave the oven on for step # 5.

4. When the eggplant and tomatoes are cool enough to handle, bring a small baking dish (about 6"x 9") and begin to assemble the Caprese salad. Arrange the eggplant, tomato, cheese and basil in the baking dish forming a tight row. Repeat the pattern until you fill the baking dish side-to-side.

5. If you like, place the baking dish in the oven to heat for 7-10 minutes (just until the cheese melts slightly).

6. While the Caprese salad warms up, make the basil vinaigrette. In a small food processor, blend the chopped garlic with the basil leaves, olive oil, lime juice and spices.

7. When ready, remove the roasted eggplant Caprese salad from the oven and spoon some of the basil vinaigrette on top. Place the extra basil vinaigrette in a bowl to serve next to the salad. Slice a loaf of crusty bread to serve along. Enjoy!

4. YOUR DINNER:

Falafel in Pita Pockets

Time - 120 m | **Servings** - 4

Ingredients:

1 cup dried chickpeas

4 cups Water

1 tsp fine sea salt

1 tbsp extra-virgin olive oil

½ tsp cumin

½ tsp coriander

½ tsp onion powder

¼ tsp garlic powder

¼ tsp fine sea salt

¼ tsp freshly ground black pepper

4 Persian cucumbers sliced

1 head romaine lettuce shredded

2 tomatoes thinly sliced

½ small red onion thinly sliced

6 whole-wheat pitas warmed and split

¾ cup tahini dressing for serving

Harissa zhoug, or sambal oelek, for serving (optional)

Directions:

1. Combine the chickpeas, water, and salt in the Instant Pot and stir to dissolve the salt. Secure the lid and set the Pressure Release to Sealing. Select the Bean/Chili, Pressure Cook, or Manual and set the cooking time for 15 minutes at high pressure. Next, select the Timer or Delay function and set the time delay for 10 to 12 hours. (When the soaking time is complete, the pot will take about 10 minutes to come up to pressure before the cooking program begins.)

2. When the cooking program ends, let the pressure release for at least 15 minutes, then move the Pressure Release to Venting to release any remaining steam. Open the pot and, wearing heat-resistant mitts, lift out the inner pot and drain the chickpeas in a colander, then transfer them to a medium bowl.

3. Add 1 ½ tsps of the oil, the cumin, coriander, onion powder, garlic powder, salt, and pepper and toss to coat the chickpeas evenly with the oil and spices.

4. Heat the remaining 1 ½ tsp oil in a skillet over medium-high heat. Add the chickpeas and sauté. for 8 to 10 minutes, until the chickpeas are slightly browned and the spices are aromatic and toasted but not burned. Remove from the heat.

5. Tuck the cucumbers, lettuce, tomatoes, and onion into the pitas, then spoon ½ cup of the warm chickpeas into each pocket. Drizzle each filled pita with 2 tbsp tahini dressing and

with hot sauce to taste. Serve the pita pockets while the chickpeas are warm.

+ YOUR DESSERTS:

Thai Red Bean Dessert

Time - 120 m | **Servings** - 5

Ingredients:

½ cup beans (red adzuki) & 1 ½ cups water

2 cans coconut milk

½ cup tapioca

2 teaspoons vanilla flavoring

½ cup sugar (or more depending on desired sweetness)

1 pinch of salt

Directions:

1. Place beans, water, salt, and seaweed (if using) in a slow cooker on "high". Cook for at least 2 hours, or until beans are soft. If more convenient, leave the beans to cook on "low" overnight or all day.

2. Once beans are soft and fully cooked, using a potato masher, mash beans into small pieces.

3. Add 1 can of the coconut milk, sugar, tapioca, and vanilla. Stir well and leave to cook on "high" for another 30 to 60 minutes. Check occasionally, adding 1 cup of water or more if the pudding becomes too thick.

4. Do a taste test for sweetness and to make sure your tapioca is cooked; it should no longer taste hard or granular. If using Asian tapioca, the "pearls" will turn transparent. Regular "minute" tapioca may take slightly longer.

5. Serve warm in bowls or dessert cups. Top the pudding with some coconut cream to create 2 distinct layers. If desired, add a sprinkling of shredded coconut and a few red jelly beans.

THANK YOU, YOU CAN DO EVERYTHING!

RECOMMENDATION:

20.A contrast shower also helps to improve health. Start with warm, then turn on cool (but not cold, and so on several times per set).

1. YOUR BREAKFAST:

Cardamom Yogurt with Roasted Peaches

Time - 10 h | **Servings** - 3

Ingredients:

8 cups whole milk

10 green cardamom pods lightly crushed

2 tablespoons plain yogurt

¼ cup granulated sugar

1 teaspoon ground cardamom

½ teaspoon vanilla extract

6 peaches halved and pitted

6 tablespoons old-fashioned rolled oats

3 tablespoons unsalted butter melted

2 tablespoons firmly packed brown sugar

¼ teaspoon ground cardamom

Directions:

1. To make the yogurt, pour the milk into the Instant Pot. Enclose the cardamom pods in a square of cheesecloth and add to the pot.

2. Lock the lid in place and turn the valve to Sealing. Press the Yogurt button until the screen says boil and cook until the milk reaches 180°F, about 25 minutes.

3. Have ready an ice-water bath. Remove the lid and check the milk temperature with an instant-read thermometer. If it is not 180°F, press the Keep Warm/Cancel program to reset the program, then select Sauté and heat until it reaches 180°F. Remove and discard the cardamom.

4. Transfer the inner pot to the ice-water bath, then stir the milk until it cools to 110°F, about 10 minutes. Transfer 1 cup of the milk to a small bowl, whisk in the yogurt until smooth, then return the milk-yogurt mixture to the pot and add the granulated sugar, cardamom, and vanilla. Whisk until blended.

5. Return the inner pot to the Instant Pot housing. Lock the lid in place; the valve can be turned to Sealing or Venting. Press the Keep Warm/Cancel button to reset the program, then press the Yogurt button and set the cook time for 10 hours. When the yogurt is ready (the screen will read Yogt), remove the lid, use pot holders to lift out the inner pot, cover it with plastic wrap, and refrigerate until the yogurt sets, about 4 hours. Do not stir at this point.

6. When the yogurt is set, line a large fine-mesh sieve with 4 layers of cheesecloth, place the sieve over a bowl, spoon the yogurt into the sieve, and refrigerate for 2 hours to drain.

7. Meanwhile, prepare the roasted peaches. Preheat the oven to 350°F. Butter a 9-inch square baking dish.

8. Arrange the peaches, cut side up, in the prepared dish. In a small bowl, stir together oats, butter, brown sugar, and cardamom, mixing well. Sprinkle the oat mixture evenly over the peaches. Roast in the oven until the peaches are juicy and tender and the topping is browned, 30–35 minutes.

9. To serve, spoon the yogurt into individual bowls and top with the peaches.

Chicken Zoodle Soup

Time - 40 m | **Servings** - 6

Ingredients:

3 stalks celery diced

2 tbsp pickled jalapeno diced

1 cup bok choy sliced into strips

½ cup fresh spinach

3 Zucchini spiralized

1 tbsp coconut oil

¼ cup button mushrooms diced

¼ medium onion diced

2 cups cooked diced chicken

3 cups chicken broth

1 bay leaf

1 tsp salt

½ tsp garlic powder

⅛ tsp cayenne pepper

Directions:

1. Place celery, jalapeno, bok choy, and spinach into medium bowl. Spiralize zucchini; set aside in a separate medium bowl. (The zucchini will not go in the pot during the pressure cooking).

2. Press the Sauté button and add the coconut oil to Instant Pot. . Once the oil is hot, add mushrooms and onion. Sauté for 4– 6 minutes until onion is translucent and fragrant. Add celery, jalapenos, bok choy, and spinach to Instant Pot. Cook for additional 4 minutes. Press the Cancel button.

3. Add cooked diced chicken, broth, bay leaf, and seasoning to Instant Pot. Click lid closed. Press the Soup button and set time for 20 minutes.

4. When timer beeps, allow a 10-minute natural release, and quick-release the remaining pressure. Add spiralized zucchini on Keep Warm mode and cook for additional 10 minutes or until tender. Serve warm.

3. YOUR SALAD:

Balela

Time - 30 m | **Servings** - 5

Ingredients:

3 ½ cups cooked chickpeas (or 2 15-ounce cans chickpeas, drained and rinsed)

½ green bell pepper, cored and chopped

1 jalapeno, finely chopped (optional)

2 ½ cups grape tomatoes (or cherry tomatoes), slice in halves if you like, or leave whole

3–5 green onions, both white and green parts, chopped

½ cup sun-dried tomatoes (use ones that have been preserved in jars with olive oil)

⅓ cup pitted Kalamata olives

¼ cup pitted green olives

½ cup freshly chopped parsley leaves

½ cup freshly chopped mint or basil leaves

For Dressing

¼ cup Early Harvest Greek extra virgin olive oil

2 tbsp white wine vinegar

2 tbsp lemon juice

1 garlic clove, minced

Salt and black pepper, a generous pinch to your taste

1 tsp ground sumac

½ tsp Aleppo pepper

¼ to ½ tsp crushed red pepper (optional)

Directions:

1. In a large bowl, mix together the salad ingredients: chickpeas, vegetables, sun-dried tomatoes, olives, and fresh herbs.
2. In a separate smaller bowl or jar, mix together the dressing ingredients: extra virgin olive oil, white wine vinegar, lemon juice, minced garlic, salt and pepper, and spices.
3. Drizzle the dressing over the salad and mix gentle to coat. Leave aside for 30 minutes before serving, or cover and refrigerate until ready to serve.
4. When ready to serve, give the salad a quick mix and taste to adjust seasoning if at all needed. Enjoy!

4. YOUR DINNER:

Mac Cincinnati Chili

Time - 60 m | **Servings** - 4

Ingredients:

Spice Blend:

1 tbsp sweet paprika

2 tsp ground cumin

1 ½ tsp ground cinnamon

1 tsp ground coriander

1 tsp natural cocoa powder

1 tsp mustard powder

½ tsp ground ginger

¼ tsp ground cloves

¼ tsp cayenne pepper

Other Ingredients:

2 tsp cold-pressed avocado oil

2 garlic cloves minced

1 yellow onion diced, plus ¾ cup chopped, for serving

1 lb 96 percent extra-lean ground beef

2 cups low-sodium roasted beef bone broth

8 oz whole-wheat elbow pasta

14 ½ oz petite diced tomatoes and their liquid one can

1 ½ cups drained cooked kidney beans or 15 oz (1 can) kidney beans, rinsed and drained

¾ cup shredded Cheddar cheese or vegan cheese shreds, for serving

yellow mustard for serving

Tabasco sauce for serving

Directions:

1. To make the spice blend: In a small bowl, stir together the paprika, cumin, cinnamon, coriander, cocoa powder, mustard powder, ginger, cloves, and cayenne.

2. Select the Sauté setting on the Instant Pot and heat the oil and garlic for 2 minutes, until the garlic is bubbling but not browned. Add the diced onion and sauté. for about 2 minutes, until it begins to soften. Add the beef and sauté. for 3 minutes, using a wooden spoon to break up the meat as it cooks. Stir in the spice blend and sauté. for about 2 more minutes, until the beef is mostly cooked through and the spices are aromatic.

3. Pour in the broth, using a wooden spoon or spatula to nudge any browned bits from the bottom of the pot. Add the pasta in an even layer, using the spoon to nudge the noodles under the liquid as much as possible. It's fine if a few pieces are sticking up out of the water. Pour the tomatoes and their liquid and the kidney beans evenly over the ground beef and pasta mixture. Do not stir them in.

4. Secure the lid and set the Pressure Release to Sealing. Press the Cancel button to reset the cooking program, then select the Pressure Cook or Manual setting and set the cooking time for 6 minutes at high pressure. (The pot will take about 10 minutes to come up to pressure before the cooking program begins.)

5. When the cooking program ends, let the pressure release naturally for 5 minutes, then move the Pressure Release to Venting to release any remaining steam. Open the pot and stir the chili mac to combine. Let sit for 5 minutes, then stir once more.

Apple Crisp Dessert

Time - 200 m | **Servings** - 6

Ingredients:

6 medium cooking apples (peeled, cored, and sliced)

1 ½ cups flour

1 cup packed brown sugar

1 tablespoon cinnamon

½ teaspoon nutmeg

¼ teaspoon ginger

¾ cup butter (softened)

Directions:

1. Generously butter the crock pot (slow cooker). Arrange apple slices in bottom of the pot.
2. In a bowl, combine flour, sugar, spices, and butter with fingers or a fork until crumbly.
3. Cover the apples with the crumble mixture. Tamp down lightly.
4. Cook on high for 3 to 4 hours or until apples are tender.
5. Serve in dessert dishes with any or all of the suggested toppings.

THANK YOU, YOU CAN DO EVERYTHING!

○ *DAY: 21*

RECOMMENDATION:

21.If you can sleep at least 20 minutes during the day, it will be very useful.

1. YOUR BREAKFAST:

Chai-Spiced Breakfast Quinoa

Time - 120 m | **Servings** - 6

Ingredients:

2 cups quinoa

5 cups Water

¼ cup honey

1 tablespoon coconut oil

2 teaspoons Ginger minced fresh

1 teaspoon ground cardamom

1 teaspoon ground cinnamon

¼ teaspoon ground cloves

¼ teaspoon ground nutmeg

¼ teaspoon salt

1 cup coconut milk refrigerated, full fat, or half-and-half

2 cups raspberries chopped strawberries, blueberries, and/or blackberries

honey topping

Directions:

1. Place quinoa in a sieve and rinse well under cool running water; let drain.
2. Combine quinoa, the water, honey, coconut oil, ginger, cardamom, cinnamon, cloves, nutmeg, and salt in the Instant Pot.

3. Secure the lid on the pot. Open the pressure-release valve. Select slow cook and adjust to more.

4. Cook for 2 to 3 hours or until grains are tender. Press cancel.

5. Stir in the coconut milk and 1 cup of the fresh berries. Top each serving with the remaining berries and drizzle with honey.

2. YOUR LUNCH:

Beef Pho

Time - 60 m | **Servings** - 4

Ingredients:

For The Broth

1 ½ pounds oxtails

½ pound beef brisket or chuck roast

1 cinnamon stick

5 whole cloves

⅛ tsp ground coriander

2 star anise pods

½ medium onion thickly sliced

2-inch piece fresh ginger thickly sliced and bruised

10 cups filtered water

½ medium fuju apple peeled and cut into chunks

2 tsp sea salt

2 tsp fish sauce or more to taste

keto-friendly sweetener (optional)

To Assemble

6 ounces sirloin steak

2 large Zucchini spiralized into thin noodles

¼ red onion thinly sliced

2 scallions thinly sliced on a diagonal

Lime wedges for serving

Toppings (Optional)

1 cup mung bean sprouts or other sprouted greens

few sprigs each of fresh thai basil, cilantro, and/or mint

thai chiles or jalapenos thinly sliced

Directions:

1. For the Broth: Rinse the oxtails and brisket well under cold running water. Place the oxtails and brisket in a large stockpot and cover with water. Bring the water to a rolling boil over high heat, then reduce to a low boil and cook for 15 minutes. You will see a beige colored raft of foam form on the surface of the water. Remove the pot from the heat, discard the water, and rinse the oxtails and brisket with warm water when they are cool enough to handle. Set the beef aside.

2. Set the Instant Pot to Sauté. Once heated, place the cinnamon, cloves, coriander, and star anise in the bottom of the dry pot insert and toast for 2 to 3 minutes, stirring constantly. Add the onion and ginger and continue to stir for an additional minute or two. The aromatics will begin to smell very fragrant during this time, and it is desirable if they begin to char slightly. Press Cancel.

3. Carefully pour in the water, then add the oxtails, brisket, apple, and salt. Secure the lid and set the steam release valve to Sealing. Press the Pressure Cook or Manual button and set the cook time to 15 minutes.

4. Meanwhile, place the sirloin in the freezer for 20 to 30 minutes (this makes it easier to slice later). Place the optional toppings in small bowls to prepare for serving later.

5. When the Instant Pot beeps, allow the pressure to release naturally for 20 minutes, then carefully switch the steam release valve to Venting. When fully released, open the lid. Very carefully strain the hot broth from the pot through a fine-mesh sieve. Set the brisket aside and discard the ginger, onion, apple, and spices. Leftover bones and cartilaginous bone caps from the oxtails can be saved and used again later to make bone broth. Season the strained broth with fish sauce to taste. Adjust the flavor by adding sweetener to taste, if desired.

6. Remove the sirloin from the freezer and slice thinly across the grain. Likewise slice the cooked brisket. Divide the spiralized

zucchini noodles evenly among four large soup bowls.
Arrange slices of both raw and cooked beef atop the zucchini
noodles, along with slices of red onion and scallion. Gently
pour a generous serving of piping hot broth into each bowl
directly over top of the raw beef slices and zucchini noodles.
Serve immediately with the optional toppings on the side for
diners to add themselves, along with lime wedges.

3. YOUR SALAD:

Eggplant Stew

Time - 8 h | **Servings** - 6

Ingredients:

2 (15 ounce) cans diced tomatoes

1 eggplant, peeled, quartered, and cut into rounds

2 yellow squash, halved and sliced

2 zucchini, cut into rounds

1 cup water

1 large onion, sliced and quartered

1 (4 ounce) can sliced mushrooms with juice

1 tablespoon extra-virgin olive oil

1 tablespoon chopped garlic

1 tablespoon dried oregano

salt to taste

Directions:

1. Combine diced tomatoes, eggplant, yellow squash, zucchini,
   water, onion, sliced mushrooms, olive oil, garlic, oregano, and
   salt in a 6-quart slow cooker.
2. Cook on Low until eggplant is tender, about 8 hours.

<u>4. YOUR DINNER:</u>

Lettuce Wraps

Time - 30 m | **Servings** - 4

Ingredients:

2 tablespoons olive oil

1 lb ground pork

2 medium carrots diced

1 bunch green onions sliced

½ cup Water

1 cup Hoisin Sauce

1 cup soy sauce

2 tsp minced ginger

½ tsp red pepper flakes

8 oz water chestnuts can, drained

1 small head bib lettuce

Directions:

1. Press Sauté button on Instant Pot. Add oil, ground pork, carrots, and green onions to Instant Pot. Cook, stirring occasionally, 5 minutes.
2. Pour in water and deglaze bottom of pot. Turn Instant Pot off.
3. In a small bowl, mix hoisin sauce, soy sauce, ginger, and red pepper flakes together. Pour sauce and water chestnuts over pork. Do not stir.
4. Close lid and set pressure release to Sealing.
5. Press Manual or Pressure Cook button and adjust time to 2 minutes.
6. When the timer beeps, allow pressure to release naturally and then unlock lid and remove it.
7. Mix ingredients together. Scoop pork into bib lettuce leaves and serve.

Hot Spiced Fruit

Time - 4 h | **Servings** - 8

Ingredients:

1 large can (28 to 29 ounces) peach slices (drained)

1 can (8 to 16 ounces) pineapple tidbits with natural juices (undrained)

1 large can (28 to 29 ounces) pear slices (drained)

1 can (15 ounces) mixed chunky fruit

½ cup maraschino cherries (drained)

1 tablespoon cornstarch

1 ½ teaspoons ground cinnamon

1 teaspoon ground nutmeg

½ cup brown sugar

4 tablespoons butter

Directions:

1. Combine all ingredients in the slow cooker; stir gently.
2. Cover and cook on LOW for about 4 to 6 hours or on HIGH for 2 to 3 hours.
3. Serve with heavy cream or a dollop of sour cream, if desired.

THANK YOU, YOU CAN DO EVERYTHING!

IV. ORANGE WEEK

22 23 24 25 26 27 28

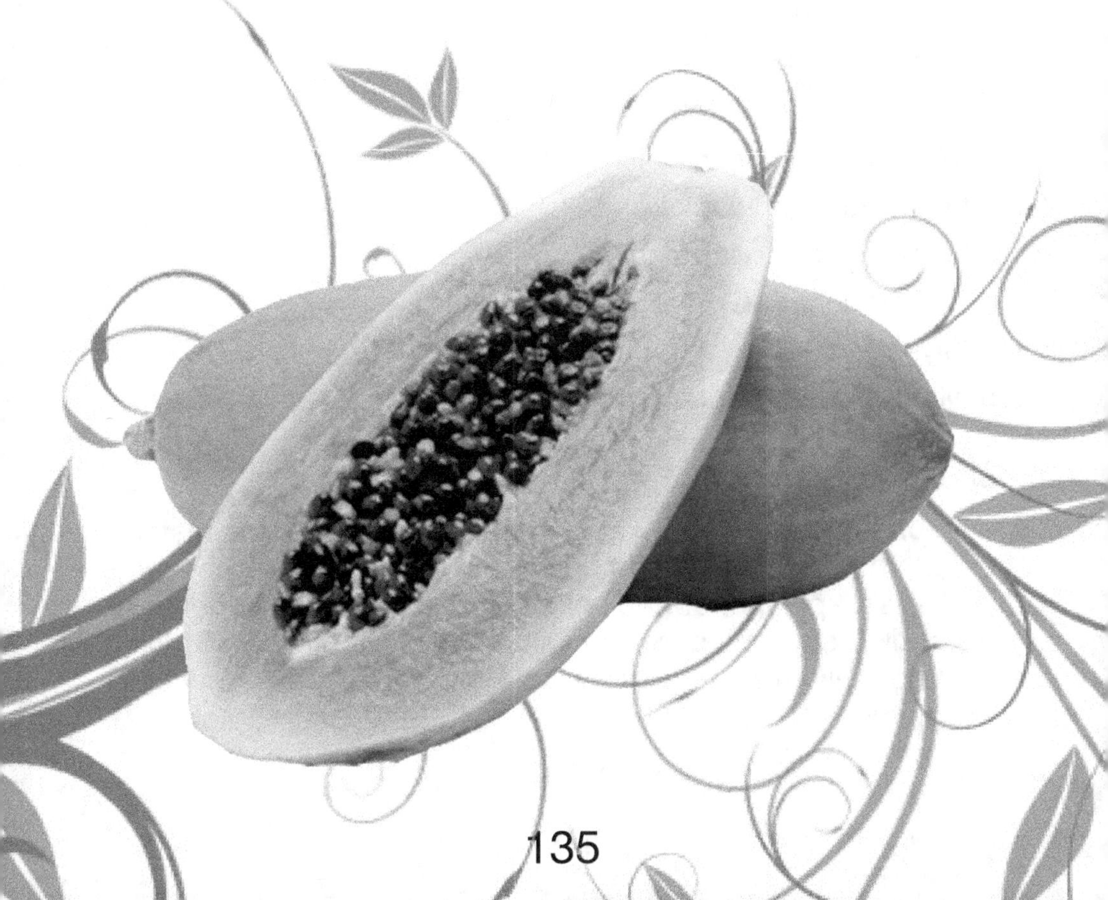

○ *DAY: 22*

RECOMMENDATION:

22. Try to reduce the amount of coffee in your diet. Over time, people become addicted to caffeine and wake up overwhelmed in the morning and only coffee brings them back to normal. It's not great, isn't it?

1. YOUR BREAKFAST:

Cheddar-Herbed Strata

Time - 40 m | **Servings** - 4

Ingredients:

6 eggs

1 cup full-fat Cheddar cheese shredded

1 cup spinach chopped

½ tbsp salted grass-fed butter softened

4 oz onion (¼ small onion) thinly sliced

½ tsp freshly ground black pepper

½ tsp kosher salt & ½ tsp parsley dried

½ tsp Dijon mustard & ½ tsp paprika

½ tsp cayenne pepper

½ tsp cilantro dried & ½ tsp sage dried

Directions:

1. Pour 1 cup of filtered water into the inner pot of the Instant Pot, then insert the trivet. In a large bowl, combine the eggs, cheese, spinach, butter, onion, black pepper, salt, mustard, paprika, cayenne pepper, cilantro, sage, and parsley. Mix thoroughly. Transfer this mixture into a well-greased, Instant Pot–friendly dish.

2. Using a sling if desired, place the dish onto the trivet, and cover loosely with aluminum foil. Close the lid, set the pressure release to Sealing, and select Manual/Pressure Cook . Set the Instant Pot to 40 minutes on high pressure and let cook.

3. Once cooked, let the pressure naturally disperse from the Instant Pot for about 10 minutes, then carefully switch the pressure release to Venting.

4. Open the Instant Pot and remove the dish. Let cool, serve, and enjoy!

2. YOUR LUNCH:

Ghee

Time - 50 m | **Servings** - 10

Ingredients:

2 lbs unsalted butter

Directions:

1. Put instant pot on sauté mode 'less'. Make sure the butter is at room temperature.

2. Put the butter in the pot and let the butter sticks melt completely.

3. Now put the instant pot to sauté mode 'normal'. The pots temperature will increase and butter will start cooking.

4. A lot of froth will come in the beginning when butter starts cooking, keep stirring occasionally.

5. Next few minutes the froth starts to reduce slowly. After few minutes the froth will be gone and white milk solids will float on top (this means that the butter is starting to get clear).

6. Keep cooking and stir occasionally, you will see that butter will get clear (yellowish golden color) and white particles get to the bottom and sides.

7. If you are looking for golden color ghee, then at this point you can turn off the instant pot. Take out the stainless steel insert

and let cool. The residual heat will further cook the ghee and the milk solids get dark golden color.

8. Once cooled, strain and store in a glass jar. (strainer, cheese cloth or coffee filters can be used). But I want caramel color to the Ghee(aka Brown butter ghee), so I will cook more time on saute mode 'less'.

9. Once the caramel color is achieved I turn off the heat and remove the stainless steel insert from the base to prevent further cooking. Store in a glass jar and cool completely overnight to get grainy solid texture.

3. YOUR SALAD:

Mediterranean Lentil Soup

Time - 6 h | **Servings** - 6

Ingredients:

18 ounces dry lentils & water to cover

½ cup olive oil & 3 carrots, sliced

1 large red onion, grated

2 tablespoons tomato paste

2 cloves garlic cloves, peeled

2 teaspoons dried Greek oregano & 2 bay leaves

Directions:

1. Place lentils in a medium saucepan, cover with water, and bring to a boil. Boil for 10 minutes, drain well, and add to the slow cooker.

2. Combine olive oil, carrots, red onion, tomato paste, garlic, oregano, bay leaves, salt, and pepper in the slow cooker and cover with about 6 to 7 cups of water. Cook on Low until lentils are soft, 6 to 8 hours.

<u>4. YOUR DINNER:</u>

Salmon with Spinach and Potatoes

Time - 20 m | **Servings** - 4

Ingredients:

1 lb small red potatoes quartered

1 cup Water

1 ¼ tsp salt divided

¾ tsp black pepper divided

4 salmon filets 5-ounces each

¼ tsp sweet paprika

½ tsp lemon zest

4 garlic cloves minced

2 tbsp avocado oil

4 cups packed baby spinach

4 lemon wedges

Directions:

1. Place the potatoes in the inner pot and add 1 cup water, ¼ teaspoon salt, and ¼ teaspoon pepper. Place a steam rack on top of the potatoes.

2. On top of the salmon add the paprika, lemon zest, ½ teaspoon salt, and ¼ teaspoon pepper and place the salmon on top of the steam rack. Secure the lid.

3. Press the Manual or Pressure Cook button and adjust the time to 3 minutes.

4. When the timer beeps, let pressure release naturally until float valve drops and then unlock lid.

5. Remove the salmon and steam rack from the pot and set aside.

6. Press the Sauté button and cook the potatoes 1 minute. Add the garlic and cook an additional 2 minutes, stirring frequently. Stir in the oil and the remaining salt and pepper.

Use a fork to gently mash the potatoes to achieve a chunky texture. Press the Cancel button.

7. Add the spinach and stir until wilted, about 1–2 minutes. Serve the salmon and potato and spinach mixture with the lemon wedges.

+ <u>YOUR DESSERTS:</u>

Tasty Rice

Time - 180 m | **Servings** - 6

Ingredients:

¾ cup long grain rice & 3 cups milk

¾ cup granulated sugar & 2 tablespoons butter

1 teaspoon vanilla extract

½ teaspoon cinnamon

¼ teaspoon kosher salt

Directions:

1. Spray the slow cooker stoneware with cooking spray.
2. Combine all ingredients in the slow cooker.
3. Cook on HIGH 2 to 3 hours or LOW 4 to 5 hours (follow the directions for your slow cooker, as they may vary depending on the model).
4. Serve warm and add toppings if desired.

<u>THANK YOU, YOU'RE A WINNER. THE BEST OF THE BEST!</u>

○ *DAY: 23*

RECOMMENDATION:

23. You can lose weight and feel better at any age, even at 70! The main desire.

1. YOUR BREAKFAST:

Hot Chocolate Breakfast Cereal

Time - 15 m | **Servings** - 4

Ingredients:

2 cups full fat coconut milk

1 cup sugar-free chocolate chips

1 cup dried unsweetened coconut

1 cup macadamia nuts

⅓ cup Swerve confectioners (or more, to taste)

¼ cup blanched almond flour

2 tbsp unsweetened cocoa powder

½ tsp cinnamon ground

½ tsp kosher salt

2 cups Water

Directions:

1. Set the Instant Pot to Sauté and add in 2 cups of filtered water, followed by the coconut milk.
2. Stir in chocolate chips, coconut, nuts, Swerve, flour, cocoa powder, cinnamon, and salt, thoroughly.
3. Close the lid and set the pressure release to Sealing. Select Manual/Pressure Cook with high pressure. The timer should be set to 0.
4. When the Instant Pot beeps, perform a quick release by carefully switching the pressure valve to Venting.

Pasta Peneer Soup

Time - 20 m | **Servings** - 4

Ingredients:

1 tbsp ghee/butter/oil

4-5 cloves garlic crushed

½ onion chopped

2 green chilies finely chopped (or adjust to taste)

1 big tomato chopped

1 tbsp bouillon paste (skip if using broth)

1 tsp garam masala (optional)

salt to taste

½ cup pasta

1 cup paneer cubes (extra firm tofu can be used as substitute)

water or broth as needed (skip if using bouillon paste)

cilantro to garnish (optional)

basil to garnish (optional)

Directions:

1. Put instant pot on Saute mode high and add ghee. Once ghee is hot add garlic and fry until aromatic.
2. Add onions and green chili, fry till edges of onions brown, then add Tomatoes and fry for 2 to 3 minutes.
3. Add Bouillon paste (skip if using broth) salt and garam masala, then add in the pasta and Paneer. Mix gently.
4. Add the water about ½ inch to 1 inch covering the pasta and mix well. (use broth if not using bouillon paste). Turn off the saute mode. Put the lid, vent to sealing position
5. Do manual (pressure cook) high 5 to 6 minutes. Let it natural release or quick release after 10 minutes in warm mode.
6. Garnish with Cilantro or basil if desired and serve hot.

Garlic Mashed Potatoes

Time - 10 m | **Servings** - 4

Ingredients:

4 medium russet yellow finn or yukon gold potatoes

1 cup vegetable broth

6 cloves garlic peeled and cut in half

½ cup non-dairy milk

Salt

¼ cup chopped parsley

Directions:

1. Cut each potato into 8–12 chunks.
2. Put into the cooker with the broth and the garlic.
3. Close the lid and turn the steam valve to "sealed"
4. Click "Manual" and reduce the time to 4 minutes.
5. When the instant pot completes the 4 minute cooking cycle, move the pressure valve to "venting" and allow the pressure valve to come down.
6. Carefully open.
7. Mash the potatoes with a masher or a hand blender.
8. Depending upon the consistency you want, add all the soy milk or not.
9. Add salt to taste and parsley and stir to combine.
10. Serve hot.

4. YOUR DINNER:

Buffalo Wings

Time - 20 m | **Servings** - 4

Ingredients:

2 pounds frozen chicken wings

½ tablespoon Cajun seasoning

1 ½ cups Water

1 cup buffalo wing sauce

Directions:

1. In a large bowl, toss chicken wings in Cajun seasoning so they are evenly coated.
2. Pour water into Instant Pot and add a trivet.
3. Place wings in a (7 inch) spring form pan. Create a foil sling and lower pan into Instant Pot.
4. Close lid and set pressure release to Sealing.
5. Press Manual or Pressure Cook button and adjust time to 15 minutes.
6. When the timer beeps, allow pressure to release naturally and then unlock lid and remove it. Remove pan from Instant Pot using foil sling.
7. Remove wings and brush with buffalo sauce. Serve hot.

+ YOUR DESSERTS:

Hot Chocolate

Time - 130 m | **Servings** - 14

Ingredients:

3 cups (about 12 oz.) powdered sugar, sifted

2 cups (about 6 ½ oz.) unsweetened cocoa

6 cups (1 ½ qt.) whole milk

6 cups (1 ½ qt.) half-and-half

2 teaspoons vanilla extract

1 teaspoon kosher salt

1 (10-oz.) pkg. dark chocolate chips (about 1 ½ cups)

Toppings: Crushed hard peppermint candies, miniature marshmal-lows

Peppermint schnapps (optional)

Directions:

1. Whisk together powdered sugar and cocoa in a 6-quart slow cooker. Turn slow cooker setting to LOW; gradually add milk and half-and-half, whisking constantly to break up lumps. Stir in vanilla and salt; cover and cook until powdered sugar and cocoa are dissolved, about 1 ½ hours.

2. Uncover slow cooker; add chocolate chips ¼ cup at a time, stirring constantly, until melted, about 2 minutes. Re-cover; continue cooking until mixture thickens, about 15 minutes.

3. Serve hot chocolate with peppermint candies, marshmallows, and, if desired, schnapps. Turn slow cooker setting to WARM to hold remaining hot chocolate up to 2 hours.

THANK YOU, YOU'RE A WINNER. THE BEST OF THE BEST!

○ *DAY: 24*

RECOMMENDATION:

24.If you decide to go to the gym, be sure to use the services of a trainer if you have no experience.

1. YOUR BREAKFAST:

Fast and Easy Shakshuka

Time - 10 m | **Servings** - 3

Ingredients:

2 tablespoons coconut oil

2 cups full-fat Cheddar cheese shredded

1 garlic clove minced

½ tsp cilantro dried

½ tsp cayenne pepper ground

½ tsp cumin ground

½ tsp oregano dried

½ tsp freshly ground black pepper

½ tsp kosher salt

14- ounce roasted sugar-free 1 can or low-sugar tomatoes

6 eggs

Directions:

1. Set the Instant Pot to Sauté and melt the coconut oil.
2. Add the cheese, garlic, cilantro, cayenne pepper, cumin, oregano, black pepper, salt, and tomatoes to the Instant Pot, and stir thoroughly.
3. Once combined, carefully crack the eggs into the mixture, maintaining the yolks. Make sure they are spaced evenly apart.

4. Close the lid, set the pressure release to Sealing, and hit Cancel to stop the current program. Select Manual/Pressure Cook , set the Instant Pot to 1 minute on high pressure, and let cook.

5. Once cooked, perform a quick release by carefully switching the pressure valve to Venting.

6. Open the Instant Pot, serve, and enjoy!

2. YOUR LUNCH:

Vegetable Sambar

Time - 40 m | Servings - 6

Ingredients:

1 tbsp oil

½ onion cubed

1 serrano pepper quartered

Salt to taste

1 big carrot diced

1 small bottle gourd diced

1 big tomato diced

1 cup yellow lentils aka toor dal or pigeon peas

1 small lime sized tamarind or concentrate 1 tbsp

½ cup cilantro

4 cups Water or as needed for desired consistency

Spices

1 tbsp red chili powder or to taste

1 tbsp coriander powder

1 tbsp turmeric

2 tbsp sambar powder

Tempering Ingredients

3 tbsp ghee (vegans can substitute with oil of choice)

7-8 cloves garlic crushed and chopped

1 tbsp mustard seeds

1 tbsp cumin seeds

1 sprig curry leaves or 10 to 15 leaves

Directions:

1. Put the pot on saute mode high, fry the seranno pepper and onions in oil. Add veggies of choice and fry for a minute.
2. Add the spices mentioned, water, lentils and tamarind extract and salt.
3. Turn off Saute mode and put manual high for 12 minutes.
4. Once natural pressure releases, check for salt and spices, boil for few mins and turn off.
5. Do the tempering and add it to the sambar, add cilantro.
6. Serve Hot with Rice and Potato chips.

3. YOUR SALAD:

Tomato & Pesto Soup

Time - 8 h | **Servings** - 12

Ingredients:

3 (14 ounce) cans vegetable broth

2 (14 ounce) cans Italian-style diced tomatoes, undrained

2 (6 ounce) cans tomato paste

3 stalks celery with leaves, chopped

2 onions, chopped

6 cloves garlic, minced

1 cup shredded carrot

1 cup water

1 teaspoon dried oregano

½ teaspoon dried thyme leaves

½ teaspoon ground black pepper

1 cup instant rice

1 (7 ounce) container pesto

⅛ cup shredded Parmesan cheese, or to taste

12 slices crusty bread, or to taste

Directions:

1. Combine vegetable broth, tomatoes, tomato paste, celery, onions, garlic, carrot, water, oregano, thyme, and pepper in a 3- to 4-quart slow cooker and mix to blend. Cover and cook on Low, 8 to 10 hours.

2. Stir rice and pesto into the cooker; cover, and let stand until rice is tender, 6 to 8 minutes. Serve soup topped with shredded Parmesan cheese and with crusty bread on the side.

4. YOUR DINNER:

Pork Tenderloin with Sriracha and Honey

Time - 60 m | **Servings** - 4

Ingredients:

1 lb pork tenderloin (or can use up to 1 ½ lbs)

2 tbsp honey & 1 ½ tsp kosher salt

2 tbsp sriracha hot sauce or to taste

Directions:

1. Insert the spit through the center of the pork tenderloin. Use a pointed metal skewer to make an initial hole if needed. Thread the rotisserie forks from each side and tighten the screws to hold the pork firmly in place.

2. In a small bowl, combine the honey, sriracha and salt. Brush evenly over the pork tenderloin.

3. Place the drip pan in the bottom of the cooking chamber. Using the display panel, select AIRFRY, then adjust the temperature to 350°F and the time to 20 minutes, then touch START.

4. When the display indicates "Add Food" use the rotisserie fetch tool to lift the spit into the cooking chamber, using the red rotisserie release lever to secure the ends of the spit. Close the door and touch ROTATE.

Pumpkin Swirl Cheesecake

Time - 10 h | **Servings** - 8

Ingredients:

1 ¼ cups graham cracker crumbs & ⅓ cup sugar

¼ cup butter, melted

2 packages (8 oz each) cream cheese, softened

¾ cup sugar & 2 eggs & ½ cup canned pumpkin

½ teaspoon pumpkin pie spice

Directions:

1. Lightly spray 8-inch springform pan with cooking spray. In small bowl, mix Crust ingredients. Press mixture in bottom and 1 inch up side of pan.

2. In large bowl, beat cream cheese with electric mixer on medium speed just until smooth and creamy; do not overbeat. On low speed, gradually beat in ¾ cup sugar, then beat in eggs, 1 at a time, just until blended. Spoon three-fourths of the cream cheese mixture into pan; spread evenly.

3. Beat pumpkin and pumpkin pie spice into remaining cream cheese mixture with whisk until smooth. Spoon over mixture in pan. Use knife to swirl cream cheese mixtures.

4. Place small ovenproof bowl in bottom of 6- or 7-quart round slow cooker (about 9 inches in diameter). Place ovenproof plate on top of bowl. Set cheesecake on plate. Place triple layer of paper towels on top of slow cooker. Cover with lid to seal. Cook on High heat setting 3 hours without removing lid. Turn slow cooker off and let stand, untouched, 1 hour. Remove cover, and transfer cheesecake to refrigerator. Refrigerate at least 6 hours before serving, but no longer than 24 hours.

THANK YOU, YOU'RE A WINNER. THE BEST OF THE BEST!

○ *DAY: 25*

RECOMMENDATION:

25.If you are too lazy or not to want to do something, you may not need to do it. Try to understand your desires and goals in life, then your path will become clearer.

1. YOUR BREAKFAST:

Classic Strawberry Jam

Time - 45 m | **Servings** - 3

Ingredients:

4 cups strawberries hulled and quartered

1 ½ cups sugar

3 tbsp lemon juice

3 tbsp Water & 3 tbsp cornstarc

Directions:

1. Mix together strawberries and sugar in the Instant Pot. Set aside for 30 minutes to allow the berries to macerate (soften and release juices).
2. After 30 minutes, add lemon juice and stir to combine.
3. Secure the lid, making sure the vent is closed.
4. Using the display panel select the MANUAL or PRESSURE COOK function*. Use the +/- keys and program the Instant Pot for 1 minute.
5. When the time is up, let the pressure naturally release for 15 minutes, then quick-release the remaining pressure.
6. Turn the pot off by selecting CANCEL , then select the SAUTE function.
7. In a small bowl, mix together cornstarch and cold water. Stir into the pot. Cook and stir until desired thickness is reached.
8. Turn the pot off and allow to cool.

Mini - Healthy Carrot Soup

Time - 20 m | Servings - 4

Ingredients:

½ medium onion diced

1 clove garlic minced

8 large carrots peeled and cut into 4-inch chunks

15 ounce can coconut milk 1 can

2 cups vegetable broth

1 teaspoon salt

½ teaspoon pepper

coconut cream for serving

chopped parsley for serving

toasted bread for serving

Directions:

1. Select the sauté function to heat the Instant Pot inner pot. When the pot displays "Hot," add the oil, onion, and garlic. Sauté until the onion softens. Press Cancel to turn off the sauté function.

2. Add the carrots, coconut milk, broth, salt, and pepper. Stir well. Secure the lid, ensuring the valve is turned to the Sealing position. Press the Pressure Cook button and set the time to 8 minutes.

3. Once cooking is complete, turn the valve to the Venting position to release the pressure. When all the pressure is released, carefully remove the lid.

4. Stir the soup. Blend with an immersion blender or in batches in a stand blender until smooth. Serve hot or cold with coconut cream, parsley, and toasted bread.

Herbed Carrots

Time - 10 m | Servings - 4

Ingredients:

1 lb fresh baby carrots or carrots cut to a similar 2 inches x ½ inch thickness

½ cup honey

1 teaspoon dried dill

1 teaspoon dried thyme

Salt to taste

2 tablespoons butter not margarine

Directions:

1. Add ½ cup water to the pressure cooker.
2. Wash the carrots and place them in a steamer tray. Place the tray in the cooker, using a cooking rack if needed to elevate it above the water level. Lock the lid in place.
3. Turn Instant Pot on to high pressure for 3 minutes.
4. Use the quick release method before opening the lid. Remove carrots and place aside for now.
5. Turn Instant Pot onto Saute Mode (medium heat) & melt the butter in . Add the dill and fry a couple of minutes or until the aroma if released. Add salt and honey, stirring to blend.
6. Add the cooked carrots and saute, turning gently until they are well coated with the honey mixture and heated through. Serve hot, spooning any remaining honey butter over the carrots.

BBQ Brisket Sandwiches

Time - 120 m | **Servings** - 6

Ingredients:

1 cup Water

3 lb beef brisket cut into ½ lb chunks

1 tbsp smoked paprika

½ cup BBQ sauce

6 sesame seed buns toasted

Additional toppings like sliced onion or pickles optional

Directions:

1. Pour one cup of water in the Instant Pot, followed by the brisket pieces. Sprinkle with smoked paprika.
2. Secure the lid, making sure the vent is closed.
3. Using the display panel select the MANUAL function. Use the +/- keys and program the Instant Pot for 60 minutes.
4. When the time is up, let the pressure naturally release for 15 minutes, then quick-release the remaining pressure.
5. Carefully remove the meat from the pot to a shallow dish and chop.
6. Stir in bbq sauce and ¼ cup - ½ cup of cooking juices to reach desired consistency.
7. Pile on toasted sesame seed buns and garnish as desired.

Plimoth Plantation Indian Pudding

Time - 120 m | **Servings** - 3

Ingredients:

3 c whole milk

½ c cornmeal

½ teaspoon table salt

2 tablespoons unsalted butter, plus extra for greasing cooker

2 large eggs

⅓ c molasses

1 teaspoon cinnamon

½ teaspoon ginger

½ c dried cranberries (optional)

Directions:

1. Grease inside of your slow cooker with butter and preheat on high for 15 minutes.

2. In a large heavy-bottom pot, whisk together milk, cornmeal, and salt and bring to a boil. Continue whisking another 5 minutes; then cover and simmer on low 10 minutes. Remove from burner and add butter. In a medium size bowl, combine eggs, molasses, and spices.

3. Add some of the hot cornmeal mixture to the egg mixture to temper the eggs; then transfer egg mixture into the pot. Stir in cranberries, if you like. Scrape batter into the slow cooker and cook on high 2 to 3 hours or on low 6-8 hours. The center will be not quite set. Serve warm topped with ice cream, whipped cream, or light cream.

THANK YOU, YOU'RE A WINNER. THE BEST OF THE BEST!

○ *DAY: 26*

RECOMMENDATION:

26. Take time to breathe. This is the foundation of our life. Often people do not breathe fully and their body lacks energy because of this. I recommend searching for Wim Hof on YouTube and studying his activities in this matter.

1. YOUR BREAKFAST:

Ace Blender - Nut Milk

Time - 120 m | **Servings** - 6

Ingredients:

warm water for soaking

1 cup nuts or seeds of choice and 47 ounces Water

Directions:

1. For best results, soak nuts or seeds in warm water for at least 1 hour, and up to 24 hours, before preparing. Drain and rinse nuts or seeds, removing any husks or skins, if desired.
2. Transfer nuts or seeds to the pitcher of the Instant Pot Ace. Fill pitcher with water to the Soup fill line (the 48 ounce)and secure lid.
3. Choose the Nut / Oat Milk program.
4. When the program has completed, filter the finished milk through the included mesh strainer bag to ensure the milk and smooth and creamy. Store refrigerated for up to 4 days.

Vegetable Kurma

Time - 30 m | **Servings** - 4

Ingredients:

1 onion finely chopped

3 tomatoes finely chopped

1 tsp Ginger-Garlic paste & 2 tsp salt

5 cups mixed veggies potatoes/carrots/beans/cauliflower/peas

1 red chili powder

2 tsp coriander powder & 2 tbsp oil

2 cups Water & 2 tbsp chopped cilantro

1 cup shredded coconut

1 tbsp poppy seeds & 1 tbsp fennel seeds

Directions:

1. Grind coconut, poppy seeds, and fennel seeds into a smooth paste adding ¼ cup of water. I used ¾ cup of water to rinse the mixer jar, and I added that to the kuruma.
2. Chop the onion, tomatoes and the veggies. You can chop the veggies roughly into chunks.
3. Set the Instant Pot in sauté mode and add oil.
4. Once the oil is hot add the chopped onions.
5. As the onions become translucent add the chopped tomatoes, ginger garlic paste, and salt.
6. Cook the tomatoes for 3-4 minutes.
7. Now add the red chili powder and coriander powder.
8. Sauté for 3-4 minutes and now add the veggies and mix well.
9. Then add the ground masala and remaining water.
10. Set the IP back to manual mode and cook for 5 minutes on a high-pressure method.
11. Let the pressure release naturally.
12. Finally, garnish it with cilantro and serve hot with Chapati.

Mashed Sweet Potatoes

Time - 120 m | **Servings** - 4

Ingredients:

2 pounds sweet potatoes, peeled and cut in 1-inch chunks

water to cover

2 tablespoons unsalted butter

1 tablespoon and 1 teaspoon milk

¾ teaspoon dried sage

¾ teaspoon salt

⅛ teaspoon pepper

Directions:

1. Place sweet potatoes in the slow cooker and add water to cover.
2. Cook on High until potatoes are tender, 1 ½ to 2 hours.
3. Place potatoes in a colander until well drained, then return to the slow cooker. Add butter, milk, sage, salt, and pepper. Mash with a potato masher until potatoes are smooth.

4. YOUR DINNER:

Oregano Scallops Alfredo

Time - 60 m | **Servings** - 4

Ingredients:

1 ¾ cups alfredo sauce 16 ouncejar

2 ½ cups chicken or vegetable broth

½ tsp dried oregano & ½ tsp garlic powder

½ tsp red pepper flakes

12 oz regular no-yolk, or gluten-free dried egg noodles

1 lb frozen bay scallops

Directions:

1. Put 1 ½ cups of the alfredo sauce in an Instant Pot. Stir in the broth, oregano, garlic powder, and red pepper flakes until smooth. Stir in the noodles, then set the block of frozen scallops right on top. Lock the lid onto the pot.

2. Option 1 Max Pressure Cooker
   Press Pressure cook on Max pressure for 3 minutes with the Keep Warm setting off.

3. Option 2 All Pressure Cookers
   Press Meat/Stew or Pressure cook (Manual) on High pressure for 4 minutes with the Keep Warm setting off.

4. When the machine has finished cooking, turn it off and let its pressure return to normal naturally for 1 minute. Then use the quick-release method to get rid of any residual pressure in the pot.

5. Unlatch the lid and open the cooker. Stir in the remaining ¼ cup alfredo sauce. Set the lid askew over the pot and let sit for a couple of minutes so the noodles continue to absorb some of the liquid. Serve hot.

+ YOUR DESSERTS:

Apple Crisp Vanilla Cake

Time - 4 h | **Servings** - 10

Ingredients:

1 can(s) (21 oz.) apple slices somewhat broken up

¼ c packed brown sugar or splenda brown sugar

½ teaspoon ground cinnamon

½ teaspoon vanilla

1 c quick-cooking oats

½ c packed brown sugar or splenda brown sugar

½ teaspoon light salt

½ c butter or light margarine: room temperature cut into small chunks

1 box yellow cake mix or sugar-free yellow cake mix

2 eggs beaten

½ c light sour cream

½ c non-fat milk or nonfat evaporated milk

⅓ c butter or light margarine, softened

½ teaspoon ground cinnamon

21 oz you can use slow-cooker stewed cinnamon apples

Directions:

1. Prepare a slow cooker with nonstick spray or grease well with margarine. In small bowl, mix apple mixture ingredients: set aside.

2. To make crumble mixture, in medium bowl, stir together oats,½ cup of brown sugar or Splenda brown sugar and the light salt. With a pastry blender or fork, cut in ½ cup of butter or light margarine until well combined. Set aside.

3. In large bowl, mix cake batter ingredients until well combined. In bottom of slow cooker, spread half of apple mixture. Top with half of crumble mixture and with half cake batter. Repeat layering again with remaining apple mixture, crumble mixture and cake batter.

4. Cover: cook on high heat setting 3 hours to 3 hours 30 minutes or until cake is set in center Turn off slow cooker. Remove cover; let stand 15-20 minutes. When reading to serve, invert coffee cake onto serving plate. Serve: With light Cool whip or vanilla sugar-free ice-cream.

THANK YOU, YOU'RE A WINNER. THE BEST OF THE BEST!

○ *DAY: 27*

<u>RECOMMENDATION:</u>

27.Massage is a very useful and enjoyable experience. But it costs money and you often need to go to special places. You can do self-massage. Just massage your back, arms, legs, face. You can do this before bedtime, then you can easily and quickly fall asleep.

1. YOUR BREAKFAST:

Mini - Blueberry-Almond French Toast Casserole

Time - 30 m | **Servings** - 4

Ingredients:

1 cup whole milk & 2 eggs

¼ cup brown sugar

½ teaspoon almond extract

½ teaspoon cinnamon

1 cup fresh blueberries or ½ cup frozen thawed

4 thick slices French bread cut into 2-inch pieces

Cooking Spray

powdered sugar for serving

slivered almonds for serving

Additional Blueberries for serving

maple syrup for serving if desired

Directions:

1. In a large bowl whisk together the milk, eggs, brown sugar, almond extract, and cinnamon until well blended. Fold in the blueberries and bread pieces until well coated.

2. Spray the baking dish with cooking spray and pour the bread mixture into the dish.

3. Place the steam rack into the Instant Pot inner pot and add ¾ cup water. Carefully lower the baking dish onto the steam rack.

4. Secure the lid, ensuring the valve is turned to the Sealing position.

5. Press the Pressure Cook button and set the time to 25 minutes.

2. YOUR LUNCH:

Lemon Cilantro Soup - Lemon Coriander Rasam

Time - 30 m | **Servings** - 4

Ingredients:

To grind into coarse paste

1 small bunch cilantro or coriander

2 tsp cumin seeds

1 tsp black pepper

2 green chili (or to taste)

1 ½ tbsp Ginger

3-4 cloves Ginger-Garlic paste

Other ingredients

1 tbsp oil

½ tsp mustard seeds

1 spig curry leaves

1 whole red chili (optional)

few pinches of Hing or Asafoetida (optional)

½ tsp turmeric powder

½ tsp toor dal (aka Pigeon peas or yellow lentils)

1 lemon juiced (or adjust to taste)

Salt to taste

water as needed for desired consistency

Directions:

1. Grind all the ingredients under "to grind" into a coarse paste without using water and keep aside.
2. Put instant pot on saute mode high and add oil.
3. Once oil is hot add mustard seeds, curry leaves, red chili, hing and turmeric powder. Fry for a minute.
4. Now add ground cilantro paste and fry for 2 minutes.
5. Now add the Toor dal and water. Along with salt. Mix well.
6. Turn off saute mode and put the lid. Vent to sealing position.
7. Do manual high 8 mins. I did natural release but you can do quick release after 5 mins in warm mode.
8. After opening the lid, check for consistency, if desired add water and put on saute mode for 2 to 3 mins.
9. Now add lemon juice and garnish with cilantro.
10. Serve hot or accompanied with rice for stir fry.

3. YOUR SALAD:

BBQ Jackfruit Sandwich

Time - 180 m | **Servings** - 4

Ingredients:

1 (16 ounce) can jackfruit in brine, drained

1 cup barbeque sauce

2 tablespoons margarine (such as Earth Balance)

4 hamburger buns, split

Directions:

1. Remove all seeds from jackfruit. Combine jackfruit and BBQ sauce in a slow cooker. Cook on High for 3 to 4 hours.
2. Use a fork to shred jackfruit meat. Spread margarine on hamburger buns and place a scoop of jackfruit "meat" on top. Serve immediately

<u>4. YOUR DINNER:</u>

Pot Pie

Time - 60 m | **Servings** - 4

Ingredients:

For the Stew:

2 cups broth of any sort

1 tbsp Worcestershire sauce

1 lb frozen ground meat. Choose from beef, buffalo, venison, pork, turkey, chicken, or even sausage meat—or a combo of any two you prefer.

2 tsp dried seasoning blend. Choose either a prepared seasoning such as Italian or Tex-Mex or a blend you create (rosemary, oregano, thyme, parsley, and basil are the norms, but enhance them with a little ground allspice or grated nutmeg).

½ tsp ground black pepper

1 lb frozen unseasoned mixed vegetables. (4-5 cups) Choose from any unseasoned blend, so long as you omit any flavoring packets. Or use a combination of frozen corn kernels, bell pepper strips, chopped onion, and/or sliced carrots.

½ cup heavy or light cream but not "fat-free" cream

2 ½ tbsp all-purpose flour

For the Biscuit Topping:

1 ¼ cups all-purpose flour & 1 ½ tsp baking powder

½ tsp table salt & 1 large egg

6 tbsp whole or low-fat milk

1 tbsp butter melted and cooled; or 1 tbsp oil of any sort you prefer

4 oz shredded semi-firm cheese. (1 cup) such as Cheddar, Swiss, or even a prepared blend, optional.

½ tsp mild paprika

Directions:

1. To make the stew, pour the broth and Worcestershire sauce into an Instant Pot. Set the pot's rack (with the handles up) or

a large, open vegetable steamer inside the pot. Set the ground meat on the rack or in the steamer. Sprinkle the seasoning blend, salt (if using), and pepper over the meat. Lock the lid onto the pot.

2. Option 1 Max Pressure Cooker
    Press Pressure cook on Max Pressure for 18 minutes with the Keep Warm setting off and the valve closed.

    Option 2 All Pressure Cookers
    Press Meat/Stew or Pressure cook or Manual on High pressure for 20 minutes with the Keep Warm setting off and the valve closed.

3. Use the quick-release method to bring the pot's pressure back to normal. Unlatch the lid and open the cooker. Use silicone cooking mitts or thick hot pads to remove the rack or steamer, letting the meat fall down into the liquid below. Use the edge of a large, metal spoon and a meat fork to break the meat up into little chunks, about the size of very small meatballs. Stir in the frozen vegetables.

4. Press the SAUTÉ button. Set it for HIGH, MORE or CUSTOM 400°F. Set the time for 5 Minutes and if necessary press START

5. Whisk the cream and flour in a small bowl until smooth. Once the liquid is simmering in the pot, add this cream mixture and whisk until bubbling. Turn off the SAUTÉ function.

6. To make the biscuit topping, stir the flour, baking powder, and salt in a medium bowl until uniform. Add the milk, melted butter or oil, and the egg. Continue stirring until the mixture has no dry ingredients in the bottom of the bowl.

7. Drop the mixture by eight blobs on top of the hot stew. Sprinkle the cheese (if using) over each of the blobs, then sprinkle each with a little paprika. Latch the lid onto the pot but do not engage the pressure valve.

8. Set the Instant Pot for SLOW COOK, set the level for HIGH and the valve must be OPEN. Set the timer for 30 minutes with the KEEP WARM setting off, and if necessary press the START button.

9. When the machine has finished cooking, turn it off and open the lid. Cool for a few minutes, then use a large cooking spoon to scoop the biscuits and stew into serving bowls.

+ <u>YOUR DESSERTS:</u>

Apples and Apricots Confiture

Time - 140 m | **Servings** - 10

Ingredients:

500 g Apples & 500 g Apricots

500 g Sugar & 1 glass Water

Directions:

1. Cut the skin from apples, but do not discard. Pour it with a glass of boiling water, place in the bowl of the slow cooker and steam in the "Steam cooking" mode for 10 minutes. This will release pectin from them, which will give perfect condensation to the future jam.
2. Catch the peel with a slotted spoon, and leave the liquid from it in the bowl.
3. Cut apples and put in the bowl of the device. Washed, seedless fruits apricots are ground in any convenient way. Spread fruit puree in a saucepan in layers, pouring sugar.
4. Cover the appliance with a lid and set the "Extinguishing" mode. Leave to languish for an hour.
5. Open the lid and mix the resulting mass. Be sure to wipe the lid from condensation.
6. Close the appliance again and set the "Baking" mode for 40 minutes. Do not close the lid tightly; in the process of languishing, mix the jam a couple of times.
7. Traditionally, lay the finished jam in sterilized jars and close it tightly.

<u>THANK YOU, YOU'RE A WINNER. THE BEST OF THE BEST!</u>

RECOMMENDATION:

28. Well, on the final day, thank yourself, you are great! I really hope that you followed at least some of my recommendations and that you feel positive changes! Good luck to you!

1. YOUR BREAKFAST:

Crustless Meat Lovers Quiche

Time - 50 m | **Servings** - 8

Ingredients:

4 slices bacon cooked and crumbled

½ cup ham diced

1 + ⅓ cup sharp Cheddar cheese shredded (divided)

2 large green onions sliced thin

6 large eggs beaten

½ cup milk

1 cup Water

Additional green onion for garnish optional

Directions:

1. Mix together the meats, 1 cup cheese and green onion in the bottom of a 1.5 quart oven-proof casserole

2. In a large bowl, thoroughly whisk together eggs and milk. Pour egg mixture over meat mixture and stir to combine. Cover loosely with foil--do not seal.

3. Pour one cup of water in the Instant Pot and insert the steam rack. Use a foil sling to carefully lower the casserole on to the steam rack.

4. Secure the lid, making sure the vent is closed.

5. Using the display panel select the MANUAL or PRESSURE COOK function*. Use the +/- keys and program the Instant Pot for 30 minutes.

6. When the time is up, let the pressure naturally release for 10 minutes, then quick-release the remaining pressure.

7. Carefully remove the casserole and top with remaining ⅓ cup cheese. Set under the broiler for 3-5 minutes until cheese begins to brown lightly. Serve immediately.

2. YOUR LUNCH:

Simle Vegetables

Time - 40 m | **Servings** - 7

Ingredients:

1-2 tbsp oil (optional)

1.5 inch piece crushed ginger

8-10 garlic crushed

½ cup cilantro tightly packed

10 mint leaves chopped

½ tsp soy sauce (or 2 tsp miso paste)

Water (see instructions for how much)

1 whole lemon juiced

VEGETABLES OF CHOICE

1 sweet onion chopped

1 carrot sliced

1 cup pumpkin pieces

1 cup winter melon pieces

2 serrano pepper

1 bunch green onion chopped

2 tomatoes chopped

½ cabbage chopped

¾ cup corn

SPICES

1 tsp black pepper

1 tsp coriander seeds

2 tsp cumin seeds

Salt to taste

Directions:

1. Put instant pot on saute mode.
2. Add oil (this is optional but gives nice flavor) and let it get hot.
3. Add ginger and garlic, fry for 2 minutes.
4. Now add all vegetables, mix well and fry for couple of minutes until they sweat and roast.
5. Add cilantro, mint and spices.
6. Add soy sauce or miso paste and mix well.
7. Add water just below the max level of Instant pot. make sure you don't exceed max level.
8. Add juice of 1 whole lemon, stir well.
9. Turn off saute mode.
10. Put the vent to sealing position, do manual 25 mins.
11. Do Natural pressure release * this is very important as there is lot of hot liquid inside, quick release is dangerous.
12. Strain the broth and can be stored in fridge for 3 to 4 days or in freezer for up to 2-3 months.

3. YOUR SALAD:

Ratatouille

Time - 4 h | **Servings** - 6

Ingredients:

6 medium zucchini, halved lengthwise and sliced

2 medium eggplants, cut into 2-inch pieces

4 yellow onions, chopped

4 medium tomatoes, chopped

3 red bell pepper, chopped

4 cloves garlic, minced

½ cup vegetable broth

¼ cup olive oil

2 teaspoons salt

2 teaspoons ground black pepper

½ teaspoon dried thyme

½ teaspoon dried oregano

Directions:

1. Combine zucchini, eggplant, onions, tomatoes, bell peppers, garlic, vegetable broth, olive oil, salt, pepper, thyme, and oregano together in a slow cooker. Cover.

2. Cook on High heat until vegetables are tender and cooked down, about 4 hours, or on Low heat for about 8 hours.

4. YOUR DINNER:

Burrito Shredded Chicken and Rice Bowl

Time - 60 m | **Servings** - 6

Ingredients:

2 tbsp extra-virgin olive oil

2 lbs boneless, skinless chicken breasts 5 - 6 chicken breasts

1 tsp ground cumin

¼ tsp cayenne pepper or taco seasoning

1 medium red or white onion chopped

4 oz green chiles chopped or diced 1 can

1 ½ cups low-sodium chicken broth

15 oz pinto beans drained and rinsed 1 can

3 cups cooked brown rice

2 medium avocados pitted and sliced, for garnish

fresh chopped cilantro for garnish

Sliced jalapeño for garnish

prepared salsa for garnish (optional)

Directions:

1. Select Sauté and add the olive oil to the inner pot. Once the oil is hot, place the chicken breasts in the pot and brown them for 2 minutes per side.

2. Press Cancel and add the cumin, cayenne pepper, onion, green chiles, and chicken broth. Using a wooden spoon, scrape up any browned bits stuck to the bottom of the pot.

3. Lock the lid into place. Select Pressure Cook or Manual; set the pressure to High and the time to 15 minutes. Make sure the steam release knob is in the sealed position. After cooking, naturally release the pressure for 10 minutes, then quick release any remaining pressure.

4. Unlock and remove the lid. Use a slotted spoon to transfer the chicken to a cutting board. Shred the chicken using two forks, and then add it back to the pot. Add the pinto beans and stir the ingredients to combine.

5. Serve immediately, or place the chicken and rice in an airtight container and refrigerate for up to 4 days or freeze for up to 2 months.

6. When ready to serve, divide the rice among six bowls and ladle the chicken mixture on top. Garnish each bowl with 2 slices of fresh avocado, cilantro, jalapeño, and a spoonful of salsa (if using).

+ YOUR DESSERTS:

Baked Apples

Time - 180 m | **Servings** - 5

Ingredients:

5 medium-sized gala apples

1¼ cups granola

3 tablespoons melted butter

5 teaspoons maple syrup

ice cream or whipped cream for serving

Directions:

1. Cut a layer off the top of the apples with a knife. With a melon baller tool, or a measuring teaspoon, remove the core and seeds from each apple.

2. Pack ¼ cup granola into each apple, and place into the slow cooker. Drizzle the apples evenly with the melted butter, and add a teaspoon of maple syrup to each apple.

3. Cover, and cook on high for 2.3 hours until tender, but not falling apart.

4. Serve as is, or add ice cream or whipped cream.

<u>THANK YOU, YOU'RE A WINNER. THE BEST OF THE BEST!</u>

The ending🩶

If your health is really important to you (both body and mind), then the foundation of this:

- *Healthy food*

- *Healthy thinking*

- *Sufficient physical activity*

- *Adequate rest (in particular sleep).*

If you debug all these 4 components, it will make you a happy person. Work on yourself with love and all the best to you. ***Be healthy and happy!***